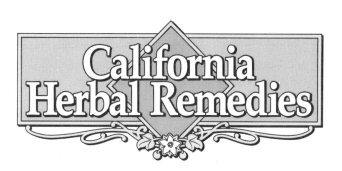

California
Herbal Remedies

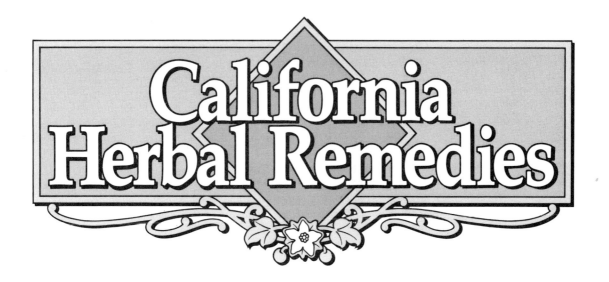

California Herbal Remedies

LoLo Westrich

Drawings by LoLo Westrich
Photographs by Jim Westrich

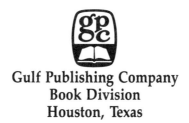

Gulf Publishing Company
Book Division
Houston, Texas

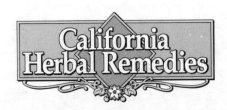

Library of Congress Cataloging-in-Publication Data
Westrich, Lolo.
  California herbal remedies/Lolo Westrich.
    p. cm.
  Bibliography: p.
  Includes index.
  ISBN 0-87201-457-6
  1. Herbs—Therapeutic use. 2. Materia medica, Vegetable-
California.
  I. Title.
RM666.H33W445   1989   89-31443
615'.321'09794—dc20   CIP

Contents

Dedicated
to
The children in my life—Joel, John, Cruz, Tyler, Dylan,
Strider, Jasmine, Holly, Alexi, and Andrew.

Acknowledgments

I am particularly grateful to these very special people for their sizable contributions to this book: my husband, Jim, not only for his fine photographs and the lengths to which he went to take them (scaling cliffs, climbing trees, rolling down hills) but for his endless patience, his valuable time, his constant encouragement, and his unwavering faith in me; to Dr. Robert Jean Vallier for all his help, his expertise and good counsel, especially for his shared insights into the world of the American Indians, their shamans, and the contents of their medicine bundles; to Dylan Gannon, for his keen eye for spotting plants that I'd never have espied without him, and for leading me to their hiding places with an excitement and zeal that matched my own.

Thanks are also due the following individuals whose personal experiences with medicinal plants have been chosen for inclusion in this book: Dorothy L. Cooper, Jean Heather Darsey, Natlee Kenoyer, Diane Kurlfinke, Casey Moneymaker, Mary Priest, Marguerite I. Reuter, and Viola Vallier.

WARNING

The information in this book is meant to add something of value to the storehouse of old western lore, to entertain, to educate, and to deepen reader awareness and appreciation of California's colorful past. The author does not intend to advise self-diagnosis, suggest the "doctoring" of others, or encourage the neglect of medical advice and treatment. Herself the daughter of a doctor, the granddaughter of a doctor, the aunt of a doctor, and the mother of a nurse, she fully respects the medical profession and is quick to urge anyone who's ill or injured to seek medical attention immediately.

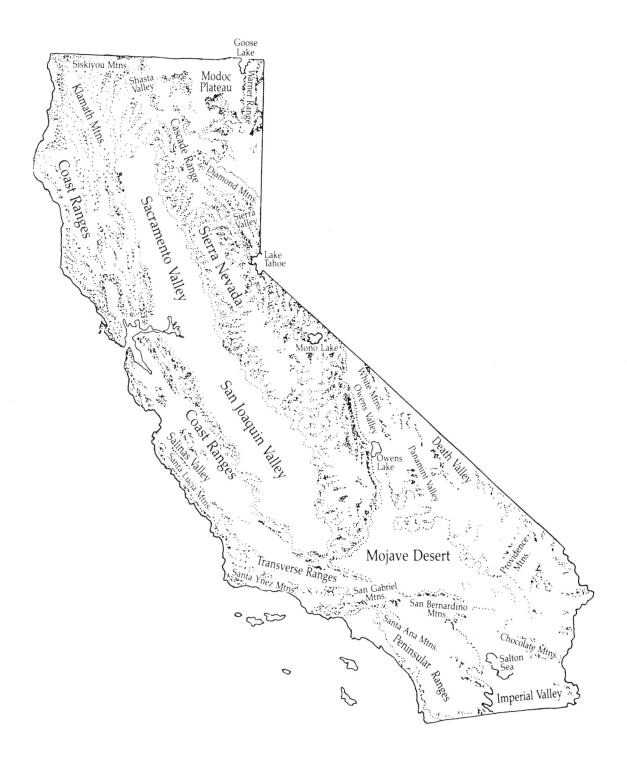

COUNTIES OF CALIFORNIA

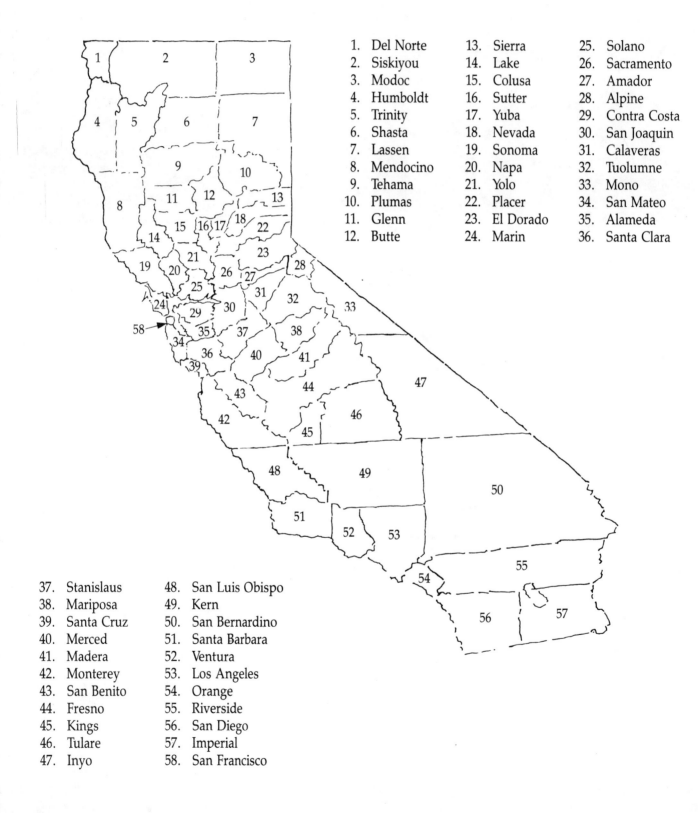

1. Del Norte	13. Sierra	25. Solano
2. Siskiyou	14. Lake	26. Sacramento
3. Modoc	15. Colusa	27. Amador
4. Humboldt	16. Sutter	28. Alpine
5. Trinity	17. Yuba	29. Contra Costa
6. Shasta	18. Nevada	30. San Joaquin
7. Lassen	19. Sonoma	31. Calaveras
8. Mendocino	20. Napa	32. Tuolumne
9. Tehama	21. Yolo	33. Mono
10. Plumas	22. Placer	34. San Mateo
11. Glenn	23. El Dorado	35. Alameda
12. Butte	24. Marin	36. Santa Clara

37. Stanislaus	48. San Luis Obispo
38. Mariposa	49. Kern
39. Santa Cruz	50. San Bernardino
40. Merced	51. Santa Barbara
41. Madera	52. Ventura
42. Monterey	53. Los Angeles
43. San Benito	54. Orange
44. Fresno	55. Riverside
45. Kings	56. San Diego
46. Tulare	57. Imperial
47. Inyo	58. San Francisco

CALIFORNIA INDIAN TRIBAL GROUP TERRITORIES

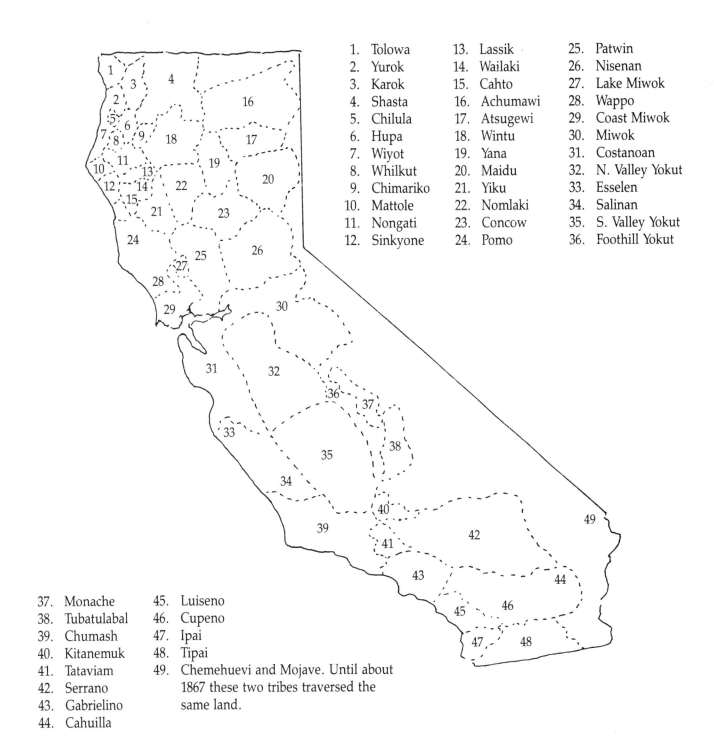

1. Tolowa	13. Lassik	25. Patwin
2. Yurok	14. Wailaki	26. Nisenan
3. Karok	15. Cahto	27. Lake Miwok
4. Shasta	16. Achumawi	28. Wappo
5. Chilula	17. Atsugewi	29. Coast Miwok
6. Hupa	18. Wintu	30. Miwok
7. Wiyot	19. Yana	31. Costanoan
8. Whilkut	20. Maidu	32. N. Valley Yokut
9. Chimariko	21. Yiku	33. Esselen
10. Mattole	22. Nomlaki	34. Salinan
11. Nongati	23. Concow	35. S. Valley Yokut
12. Sinkyone	24. Pomo	36. Foothill Yokut

37. Monache	45. Luiseno
38. Tubatulabal	46. Cupeno
39. Chumash	47. Ipai
40. Kitanemuk	48. Tipai
41. Tataviam	49. Chemehuevi and Mojave. Until about
42. Serrano	1867 these two tribes traversed the
43. Gabrielino	same land.
44. Cahuilla	

After David L. Fuller, *California Patterns, A Geographical and Historical Atlas*, Mayfield Publishing Co., 1983.

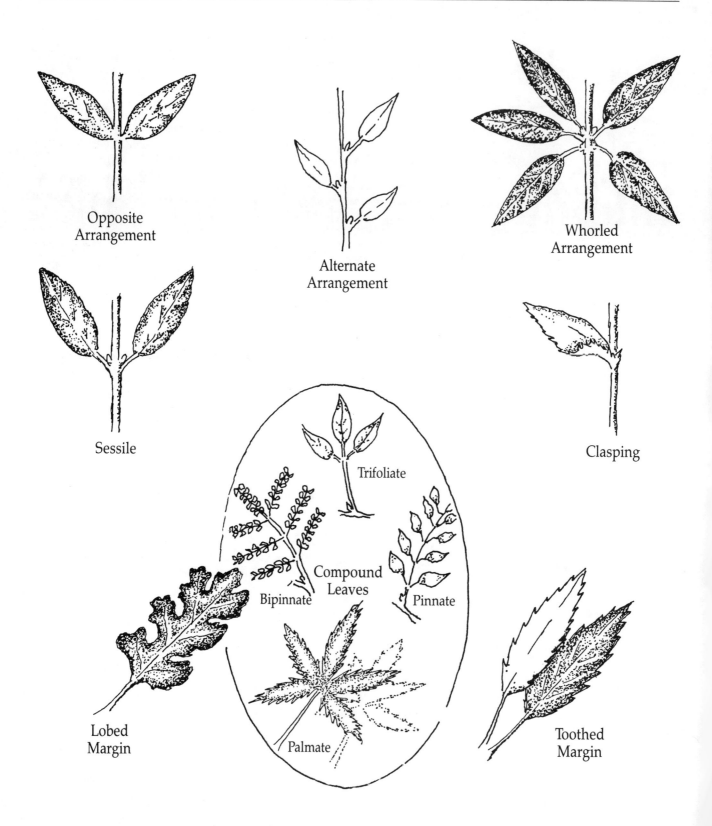

Opposite
Arrangement

Alternate
Arrangement

Whorled
Arrangement

Sessile

Clasping

Trifoliate

Bipinnate

Compound
Leaves

Pinnate

Lobed
Margin

Palmate

Toothed
Margin

1
Introduction: California Folk Medicine—Cross-Purposes in Paradise

From Angelica to Red Pepper, from the chants of shamans to the potions of mission padres, from the miners' strong, black coffee to the yeoman's blistering mustard plasters, there's no more colorful lore in our fifty states than that of the folk medicine of California. In a sense this seems odd, for here's a land that's been so roundly hailed for so many decades as one of the healthiest in America, that the words "California Folk Medicine" read almost like a contradiction in terms.

Even when it was still thought to be an island and was depicted as such on the maps of the day, California was credited with a salubriousness only Eden could match. People had been primed to see it this way. After all, it was the namesake of a wondrous mythical land, dreamt up and put on paper by an inventive sixteenth-century Spaniard by the name of Garci Rodriguez Ordonez de Montalvo. "Know ye," that gentleman wrote, doubtless with tongue in cheek, "that on the right hand of the Indies there is an island called California, very near the Terrestrial Paradise." He went on to describe a place peopled with Amazon-like women, a land where the only metal to be found was gold.

Of course, Montalvo's credibility was doomed to be shattered, as was that of the cartographers who later depicted this namesake of his dreamland as an island. Yet it's as if that alluring designation, "very near the Terrestrial Paradise" was to leave its mark. It did seem to fit the real California remarkably well. Wasn't the mountain air bracing here, the sea breeze tonic, the clime of the land as mild as a mother's smile? And didn't this all add up to a promise of verve and good health? Certainly to all those who set foot in California in its halcyon days "yes" was the unqualified answer to questions like these.

Yes, said the the young Spanish scientist, Jose Longinos Martinez, who traveled to California in 1792 to learn all he could of its phenomenal flora and fauna. In those days the land still resounded with the roars of grizzly bears. Indians accustomed to stalking their enemies moved stealthily through the woods. Hazards lurked around every corner, but Martinez unabashedly declared, "This country is among the most healthful that I have visited."

Decades later, shortly before the gold rush, similar testimony flowed from the pen of the ailing journalist Edwin Bryant who came to California for the specific purpose of regaining his vigor. He wasn't disappointed. "I never felt while there the first pang of disease," he happily recalled, "or the slightest indication of bad health."

Equally glowing were the claims of William Heath Davis, Jr., boy merchant from Hawaii who came to ply his trade in this promising land in the 1830s, when the tolling of the mission bells still ushered in each new day. Years later, he was to express his ongoing awe over the longevity of the Spanish Californios he'd come to know. According to his testimony, "in Monterey, the capital under the Mexican regime, there are still living (1889) a number of women of Castilian extraction who are ninety years old and upward."

It's true that the old-time Californians did seem to be a breed apart. From tooth to foot, they were remarkably fit. The Spanish settlers (the "Californios," as they called themselves), for example, could drink hot chocolate every morning, nibble on panoche (hard sugar) all day long, chomp on a piece of Don Pico's home-grown sugar cane whenever they could get it—do all this and yet never have a cavity, never lose a tooth, apparently never even suffer from sugar overload. And as to their feet, these were so tireless, so supple and strong that even the old folks could dance the fandango all night long. It was little wonder that those who saw them or knew them felt almost beholden to sing the praises of the land that had bred them.

Nonetheless, California's early propagandists never meant to convey the impression that people sojourning in this land didn't suffer their share of physical vexations. On the contrary, they sometimes dwelt upon their own discomforts at considerable length. Bryant, for example, verged on hyperbole as he described his adventures with the fleas that infested his bedroll. Of a few hours in the company of the latter he wrote "if any sinning soul ever suffered the punishments of purgatory before leaving its tenement of clay, those torments were endured by myself last night. When I rose from my blankets this morning, after a sleepless night, I do not think there was an inch-square of my body that did not exhibit the inflammation consequent upon a puncture by a flea, or some other equally rabid and poisonous insects. Smallpox, erysipelas, measles, and scarlet-fever combined, could not have imparted to my skin a more inflamed and sanguineous appearance."

The prominent early settler, John Bidwell, was another gentleman who could speak from experience regarding California's superabundance of blood-sucking parasites. Shortly after his arrival in 1841 he was unceremoniously locked in jail at the Mission San Jose (all because he lacked a passport, which, incidentally, he'd gone there to obtain) and hence spent three torturesome days confined in a dank cell where "the fleas were so numerous as to cover and darken anything of a light color."

Apparently bedroll-invaders were such an enormous problem in the land that, even had there been no other ills to contend with, the beleaguered humans would have felt called upon to concoct salves, ointments, or repellants of some sort just so they could cope with the insects.

But there *were* plenty of other complaints to reckon with, some of them much more serious than the ravages of fleas. For all his glowing reports about good health and good weather, the Spaniard, Martinez, took care to note some tragedies as well. "Many Indians die also from snakebite," he noted. "Sometimes those who have been bitten are cured with remedies, but most of them die more or less speedily." And elsewhere he grimly commented that syphilis was making "rapid headway among the Indians, more than among the settlers, and in time they will become victims of this virus, as has happened in Old California, unless some remedy is provided for it." Bryant wrote of the malaria that was spreading so perniciously in the interior riverlands when he visited there in the 1840s. Even the generally-undespairing Davis admitted that he himself was ill for many of his California years, that he was afflicted with chronic "neuralgia in the head" and was, in fact, "on the point of death," until another resident, a Spanish lady by the name of Dona Guadalupe, treated him with a "simple remedy" (the nature of which, regrettably, he did not divulge) that cured him forever.

The truth is that, like any place else short of Paradise, California was not without a fair allotment of woes and vexations. Of course, there were always those so determined to believe that it *was* Paradise that they chose to ignore this fact, to insist it wasn't so, to pretend that every illness and every tragedy was only an anomaly. Such a person, apparently, was a certain forty-niner by the name of Peter Decker, a stick-to-it-ive young man who wrote in his diary that disease was "seldom fatal in this country" in the very same sentence in which he also recorded the death of two cohorts struck down with cholera.

It's fair to say that people who lived in frontier California were more robust than people living elsewhere, that Californians recovered faster when they were ill, and stayed well longer. But on the other hand, here in this "terrestrial Paradise" the hazards were more extreme; hardships were many; more wild beasts marauded; store-bought medicines were hard to get; and doctors were so few as to be discounted. Here, as elsewhere, people caught colds, suffered from rheumatism, got bitten by snakes, broke their bones, and were plagued by insects. Mothers gave birth, babies cried, youngsters coughed, and the cholera spread. Here too, the residents fashioned their own compendium of folk cures and remedies to which they turned to make their lives in a truly wild frontier more tenable. But what an uncommonly variegated and ever-changing bundle of regional lore it was. It had to be. It had to fit the needs and tastes and backgrounds of a conglomorate of cultures that ranged from that of Indians, whose ills were sometimes seen as frog-like, living entities that had invaded their bodies, to Spanish senoras seeking fountains of fertility; from yeomen concocting snakebite potions, to erudite New Englanders with medical books in their saddlebags.

To know California's old-time remedies is to know the land, its flora, its fauna, its wilderness, its parks, people, towns, and its history in a most intimate way.

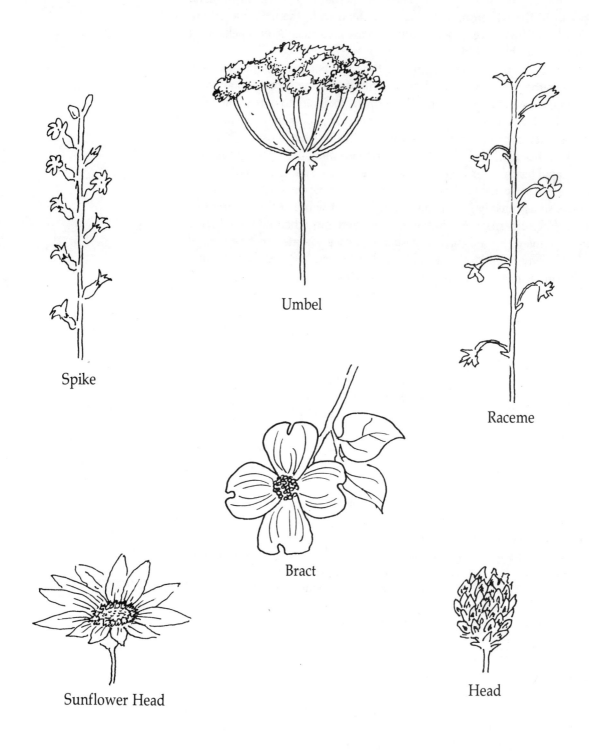

Spike

Umbel

Raceme

Bract

Sunflower Head

Head

FLOWER ARRANGEMENTS

2
Old Remedies that Grow Wild in California: A California Herbal and Field Guide

ALDER

Alnus spp.

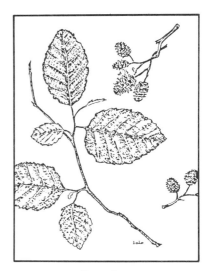

Red Alder

Other names for the Alder: English names for the various species of Alder are Red Alder, White Alder, Sitka Alder, and Thinleaf Alder. The Yuki Indian name for their favorite Alder was *Um-se*. The Wailaki called theirs by two names: *Jus-ki-at* and *Kus*. To the Pomo the Alder was *Ga-shet*.

Where to find it: You'll find this handsome but short-lived hardwood growing in moist places, sometimes flourishing by the sides of streams, often in the company of other moisture-lovers, like the Big Leaf Maple Tree, the willows, and the cottonwoods; and other thirsty wildings.

In some of its habitats—for example, along Whitewater Creek in the desert near Palm Springs—these rapid-growing trees form thickets so lush they're veritable jungles.

How to know it when you see it: If it's springtime and you come across a thicket that bears a cast of greenish-brown so pronounced it's almost as if you're viewing it through dark glasses, you've probably stepped into the realm of the handsome Red Alder. It's the catkins that hang from these trees like a convention of brownish caterpillars—actually its flowers—that lend the woods this rustiness.

Alders have leaves that are prominently veined, and distinctly toothed, "exactly the way a leaf should look," as one new medicinal-plant enthusiast so aptly put it. Those of the Red Alder's are dark green above, lighter on the underside, while the White Alder's are smaller, velvety, and lighter green, a pleasing sight to see when the summer sun comes filtering through the branches.

These fast-growing, short-lived moisture lovers bear small cone-like strobiles, reminiscent of miniature pinecones, that often find their way into the pockets of children roving through the woods.

Its lore. In 1792, when the Spaniard named Jose Longinos Martinez came to California to learn its natural secrets, he listed the Alder among five important trees that grew here abundantly. He didn't mention its medicinal uses, but it's hardly likely they escaped him, for he was keenly interested in the folk medicine of the Indians, and to those native Californians the Alder was the source of many a remedy, many a cure.

One of its species, the lovely White Alder, was a stand-by medicament of several northern tribes, such as those who dwelt in what is now Mendocino County, where the tree grew so profusely around every random source of water that most any gurgling freshet there came to be known as an "alder spring."

This tree was a true heal-all, widely praised as a producer of perspiration, a purifier of blood, a cure for diarrhea, a boon for stomach aches, a facilitator of childbirth, and a treatment for the hemorrhages of consumptives. Even as late as the early twentieth century, many native Americans still swore by a decoction made from its bitter-tasting bark.

It was not only the Indians, however, who valued the Alder as a medicine. So too did the early white settlers who came to be their neighbors. If they didn't know of its usefulness already, they were quick to learn from the Wailakis and the Yukis, who were apparently willing to share their recipes for healing decoctions.

But chances are the tree's reputation wasn't news to them at all, for herbalists down through the decades had been expounding its virtues. Its bark could serve as a substitute for quinine; decoctions made of it could lower a fever, ease an ache, cure a pain; its leaves, when placed in the shoes of a weary traveler, would cool and soothe his burning feet; a solution of vinegar, in which a bit of bark had been simmered and steeped at length, was a useful lotion for combatting scabies or mites and other vexing itches.

Today most of the old Alder remedies belong to the past, as surely as do the people who took them to heart with so much zeal and confidence. Nowadays this tree, once used to heal and soothe and salve, is appreciated most for its ability to establish itself quickly in burned or logged-off land and for the way it has of adding much-needed humus and nitrogen to the soil in these places, rendering it healthier for all else that grows, including the more economically valuable conifers.

AMOLE

Chlorogalum pomeridianum

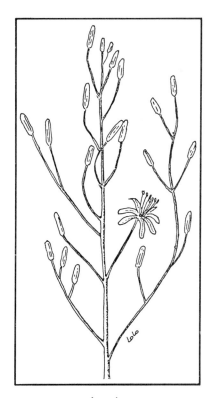

Amole
(Soap Plant)

Other names for the Amole: Other popular English names for the Amole are Soap Lily and Soap Plant. It is believed that the Cahuilla Indians called this plant *Mocee*. To the Yuki it was *Nosh*, to the Wailaki it was *Gos-cha*, to the Numlaki, *Shla*, and to the Pomo *Am*.

Where to find it: Amole is found on dry hills and plains, in open woods, and on the rocky banks of creeks and streams from Oregon to southern California. The rugged banks of Mark West Creek in Sonoma County are a haven for this once-utilitarian wilding.

How to know it when you see it: It isn't always easy to identify this fascinating wild medicinal, especially when the sun is hot and the skies are bright , for the dainty little flowers of the Indians' beloved Amole keep themselves secret until late afternoon or early evening. Be on the lookout for a spindly-looking stem that rises up from the earth lone and leafless but freely branched at the top and bearing there a number of slender pedicels. Each of these is graced with what appear to be tiny capsules shaped like infinitesimal watermelons—actually flower buds curled up and waiting for the hour of their debut. If it's *Chlorogalum pomeridianum* that you've found, you may see a large basal rosette of wavy-edged linear leaves at the foot of the long stout stem. If instead you've stumbled on *Chlorogalum angustifolium*, the leaves you'll sight will lack that waviness. In either case, don't go away. Or if you do, then come back later, just before the sun goes down. The Amole flowers—here tonight, gone tomorrow—are well worth waiting for.

Its lore. It would be audacious to say that the Indians never sought out Amole for so impractical a purpose as watching its little lily-like flowers open up to the moon. The native Californians loved the flora in a way incomprehensible to those of us who were born and bred to four walls. They ate flowers; they healed with flowers; they saw each flower as an entity (as surely as they thus saw the bear or the deer or the squirrel who vied for their acorns); some of them, such as the home-loving Maidu, perceived of heaven as simply "Flower-land." So it may well be that they hovered about the lone-stemmed soap plant in wonder sometimes, just to see its time-clocked buds uncurl. But that's not all they did. They dug up the big, deeply-buried, and hirsute bulb of the plant to use as a soap, as a richly lathering cure for dandruff, a boon to the scalp. (Even in the early twentieth century some old squaws declared it was a better cleanser than any on the shelves of the white man's store.) The Wailakis rubbed its raw juice on the body to ease away cramps or the pains of rheumatism; they roasted the root and used it antiseptically as a poultice for stubborn sores; they devised a decoction of it to use as a diuretic and a laxative, and for gas in the stomach. The Patwins of the San Francisco Bay region used an extract of Amole as an external rub, which they applied to their distended bellies when their stomachs were bloated from eating too much raw clover.

Naturally such a useful plant was bound to strike the fancy of newcomers to California. Some Americans, like Kentucky journalist Edwin Bryant, who came to California before the gold rush, were so enthralled by its properties that they gave it considerable mention in their writings. "The botany and flora of California are rich, and will hereafter form a fruitful field of discovery to the naturalist," wrote Bryant. "There are numerous plants reported to possess extraordinary medical virtues. The 'soap plant' (Amole) is one which appears to be among the most serviceable. The root, which is the saponaceous portion of the plant, resembles the onion, but possesses the quality of cleansing linen equal to any 'oleic soap' manufactured by my friends Cornwall & Brother of Louisville, Ky."

Some newcomers even devised uses for the Soap Plant that had apparently been unknown to the natives. According to V. K. Chestnut, who made a study of Round Valley's plant usage in the late nineteenth and early twentieth centuries, it was a white settler who taught an Indian that the soapy juice of this peerless bulb was a good lotion for the cure of Poison Oak.

The Amole plant served other than medicinal purposes too. Sometimes it was a nutritious food: the young shoots, deliciously edible, were as sweet as sugar when roasted. Sometimes the juice of the cooked bulb served as glue that securely attached feathers to the arrows they graced. Or the crushed parts of the entire plant were used for the purpose of stupefying fish—the better to catch them and eat them for dinner along with the sweet roasted shoots that the youngsters relished. But the medicinal, cleansing, and cosmetic purposes of this remarkable kin of the lily were the most important. Its second name was "Soap Plant," and so it remains.

ANGELICA

Angelica spp.

Other names for the Angelica: Other common English names for Angelica are Alexander's Angelica, Bellyache Root, Wild Celery, Archangel, Dead Nettle, Aunt Jericos, Root of the Holy Ghost. To the Pomo and Yokia Indians this plant was called *But-cho-a*. To the Yuki it was *Chi-en*. The Spanish Californios called it *Osha del Campo*.

Where to find it: Angelica thrives in low rich loam and in shady places, often close to running streams. See it in water-fed ravines, on wooded slopes, in damp meadows and marshes, on banks of brooks, and on coastal bluffs or flats sometimes only a stone's throw away from the sea.

How to know it when you see it: Look for a robust herb with thick hollow stems that can grow as high as six feet; a hefty-looking plant with an umbel of whitish flowers best described, perhaps, as "a ball of balls." One species, *Angelica Hendersonii*, grows rampantly along the Northern California coastline right on the shoulders of winding roads, or even in tourist-packed parking lots, and has an almost fat and overstuffed look about it, like a plant someone conceived of in kindergarten.

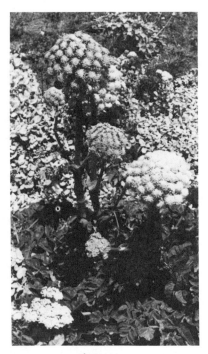

Angelica

Angelica's broad hollow stems are sinewy and succulent. Don't expect to reach over and snap one off. Twist it or bend it; even wring it like washcloth, and it still won't break loose. Yet, oddly enough, if you pull it from the top the entire plant is easily uprooted. If you're a novice to the world of the wildings don't hasten to handle any of California's umbelled plants. It's a sorry fact, but Angelica, perhaps the most beloved of all the old California cure-alls, is easily confused with certain deadly poisonous members of the carrot family, culprits responsible for many an accidental death.

Its lore. To the California Indians, there was no more beneficent herb in all the land than the versatile Angelica, for here was a plant that could heal the body, soothe the mind, fill the belly, and even please the spirits that ruled the world and made the fish run. During the most moving part of the salmon ceremony, when the Karoks convened to set the world aright, it was Angelica Root that was thrown into the fire as an offering to please the gods and ensure good angling. The shamans of almost every tribe made frequent use of the herb. Even in cases when chanting or dancing or suction or massage was the principal method of treatment, this herb usually played some important role in the cure of every patient. With some tribes, like the Hupa of the Lower Trinity, who danced and prayed much more than they warred, it was virtually the only medicinal plant that their physicians used. With such a prized panacea, apparently they needed no other.

The Pomo and the Yokia and the Yuki were not so singleminded. Like the white settlers, they cherished many herbs and their list of remedies was long and colorful. Yet, significantly enough, none ranked higher in their eyes than the Hupa's prized cure-all; none other was so bound up in wonder and magic. Even as late as the early 1900s, Angelica Root was found in nearly all their households. Sometimes it was carried about the person for good luck, like a rabbit's foot or an amulet that could make things go well in gambling or hunting or other pursuits that were otherwise left to chance. Old-timers claimed that a little chunk of Angelica root was every bit as powerful a talisman as it was a medicine. And, of course, no one ever doubted its medicinal prowess. Mashed up, it was rubbed on the bare legs to ward away venomous snakes. It was chewed and swallowed as a remedy for colic and fever. For catarrh and for colds it was crushed and smoked like Indian tobacco. Its juice, combined with saliva, was used as a treatment for sore eyes. Crushed or ground-up, it was tied about the head and ears to ease away a headache or an earache or—unlikely as it seems—to prevent nightmares.

White settlers, too, took Angelica into their hearts and into their medicine larders. Many of them had been using one species of the herb or another even before they'd come to California, having learned about it from Indians back east, or perhaps from their own family herbals, where Angelica was surely listed along with homey recipes for an assortment of tisanes, syrups, liniments, and salves with which they could treat their ills. If they'd been schooled by redskins they probably drank an Angelica tonic whenever they were convalescing. To treat arthritis, pluerisy, pneumonia, sore throats, and common coughs they may have mashed the roots and applied the resultant mushy glob to the affected body parts. Or they sipped a long-steeped root tea to cure bad breath, treat kidney trouble, soothe stomach ulcers, calm heartburn, ease sour stomach, combat tuberculosis, or even to counteract the ravages of venereal disease.

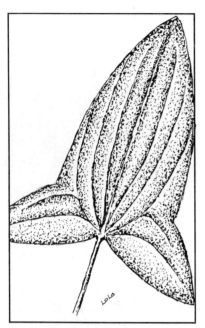

Arrowhead

ARROWHEAD

Sagittaria latifolia

Other names for the Arrowhead: Other common English names for this plant are Duck Potato, Swan Potato, Swamp Potato, Tule Potato and Marsh Potato. The Pomo Indians called it *Tsu-ish*.

Where to find it: This handsome water-lover is commonly seen in fresh-water marshes, at the edges of ponds, in meadows, in slow streams, and shallow lakes over much of California. Often its habitat is also that of the Red-winged blackbird. Listen for a song that sounds like windbells moving in the breeze and you just might be in the right vicinity to spot an Arrowhead plant.

How to know it when you see it: If you're lucky and the specimen you've spotted is a classic one, then its large leaves are shaped so much like its namesake, the Arrowhead, that you wouldn't need a field guide to guess its identity. In this case its most common moniker is a perfect clue to the looks of this widespread herb. But as it happens, the leaves of *Sagittaria* differ greatly, not only from plant to plant, but on single plants as well. Some are absolutely arrowhead-shaped; some are lancelike. Others—such as those that have been growing a long time submerged—look like so many hair ribbons twining in the water. But don't give up. You can still identify this aquatic wonder. The leaves, whatever their width, have parallel veins that are variable in width. The flower stems are smooth, wand-like, and leafless. At their tips are their lovely white flowers, which bloom from June to September, three-petaled, in whorls of three, bearing numerous pistils and yellow clusters of stamens.

Its lore. As sure as clockwork, as sure as the rise and fall of the coastal tides, every autumn before the coming of the twentieth century found the Indian women of California sloshing about in the ponds and lakes and marshes, on their way to harvest the tubers of the wonderfully edible, blessedly medicinal Arrowhead plant. Laughing, pushing their canoes before them, they loosened with their practiced bare toes the bank-bound roots of their booty. They pulled and tugged until up came the muddy treasure, right to the surface, ready to be plopped into their baskets and taken home.

Tubers harvested in this manner, or those loosened with prodding sticks instead of wiggling digits, often served later as a tasty meal, slow-baked in burning embers. But they were also a popular remedy, especially to the white settlers, influenced as they were by certain writers of the day, who believed that the juices of the Arrowhead tubers increased the flow of urine, released harmful wastes from the body, and helped to restore health to the weak and the ailing.

Except for an occasional survivalist, or an herbalist who fancies the old neglected cure-alls, the "tule potato" has long since fallen into disuse. It's definitely harmless; it's certainly edible; it's probably nutritious; it *may* even have helped the old-timers stay sound of body. Yet nonetheless, nowadays it's almost forgotten. It's as much a part of yesterday as an Indian woman wading up to her neck in icy water, reaching for muddy roots with her agile toes, while her dark-eyed youngsters watch her from the bank.

BARBERRY

Berberis repens

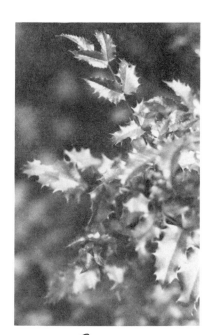

Barberry

Other names for the Barberry: Other popular English names for this plant are Oregon Grape, Mountain Grape, Dragon Grape, Mountain Holly, American Barberry, California Barberry, Common Barberry, Jaundice Barberry, Blue Barberry, Creeping Barberry, Sourberry, Wood Sour, Sowberry, Yellow Root, Pepperidge Bush, and Creeping Barberry.

Where to find it: You'll come across Barberry sometimes in mixed evergreen forests, keeping company with other wildings like Huckleberry, Hazelnut, and Salal. It thrives too on rocky hillsides, in sleepy pastures, by fences and walls, and sometimes right by roadsides where it's easy to spot when you're driving by.

How to know it when you see it: Sometimes spiny, sometimes unarmed, Barberry is a common bush-like herb that grows up to twelve feet tall in mountainous regions through most of California. Sometimes its grey-tinged branches are slightly weeping, as if they're weary from the weight of their own twigs and leaves. The wood and inner bark of the plant is golden, and so too, most often, are the fragrant flowers that hang in drooping clusters in the spring of the year. Each of these aromatic blossoms is about one quarter inch in diameter.

The leaves of the Barberry, sharply toothed, shaped like those of holly, are gleaming masses of the liveliest green in the summertime, but even then they flick and flash shades of mouse-gray when their backsides are exposed in a quickened breeze. They're changelings, masters at the art of prestidigitation. In the fall, oxidized, they sport shades of yellow, russet, brown, and the purest crimson, a tribute to the season, a delight to the eyes.

As to the fruit of this prized old medicinal, depending on the species, it runs the gamut from an almost fire-engine red to a deep lenten purple.

Its lore. Those herbalists who still cling to a comforting old school of thought called the Doctrine of Signatures must nod knowingly at the mention of this colorful shrub. According to their belief, long-outdated though it is, every single medicinal plant on the face of Mother Earth comes bearing a sort of "signed statement," as it were, which plainly reveals its potential uses to whoever takes the time to read it. So it goes with the Barberry. Its golden wood (from which the pious Spaniards used to fashion crucifixes) is quite plainly its signature. It's the yellowest of golden yellows; yellow is the tint of jaundiced flesh; hence, here's an herb meant to treat an ailing liver.

Although it was frowned upon by the burgeoning scientists of the nineteenth century, the Doctrine of Signatures was still so popular with ordinary people that the early settlers called this yellow-wooded plant the "jaundice berry bush." This is not to say that liver complaints were all they used it for, however. Far from it. They took it for constipation, for chronic coughs, stomach upsets, spleen derangements, choleric humours, ringworm, diarrhea, bloody flux, itching, bronchial trouble, poor appetite, fevers, scurvy, and general run-down conditions like spring fever or the love-sick blues.

The California Indians may never have heard of the Doctrine of Signatures but they knew, through centuries of trial and error sampling, the purpose of each and every plant whose habitat they shared. Some of these wildings—like Barberry, which afforded them berries from which to make preserves, fibers to weave into their baskets, dye to color those contrivances, and good medicine to heal their ills—were so blessedly multipurpose they were almost as much a part of their lives as prayer and dance.

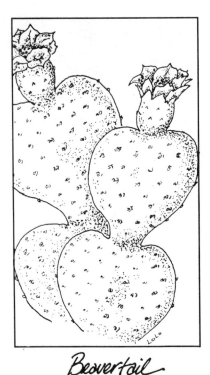

Beavertail

BEAVERTAIL

Opuntia basilaris

Other names for the Beavertail: Beavertail Cactus, Beaver Cactus, Beavertail Opuntia. The Cahuilla name for this plant was *Manal*.

Where to find it: There's as much variation in this fine native species of cactus as there is in its habitat, and its range is notably far and wide. It's at home in creosote bush scrub, in Joshua Tree woods, on the Mohave and Colorado deserts, on dry benches and fans below 6,000 feet in many locations throughout the state.

How to know it when you see it: Beavertail is a very distinctive form of cactus, flat-jointed, low-spreading, spineless—but not without some very wicked weaponry of its own. It's covered with long sharp hairs (spicules) capable of penetrating the flesh and causing considerable pain. These render it much more difficult to handle than it is to identify.

The joints of Beavertail are often remarkable for their color, ranging from white-washed green to soft grayish-lavender. The elegant rose or fuchsia-colored flowers, which bloom from March to June, look as if they're carved from wax by an artist with a delicate touch.

Its lore. To the Indians, especially those in Southern California, there was no more important cactus than the *Opuntia basilaris*. These enterprising natives used the fruit and flower buds and even some of the young fleshy joints as a foodstuff. It was tedious to prepare , yet tasty and nutritious, well worth the time it took to ready it for mealtime. But it was the older pads that served as medicine. Their pulp provided a peerless wet dressing for bruises and sores, bites and lacerations, an application said to deaden pain and hasten healing. In a time and place when sterile gauze and Band-Aids were unknown, the natives would have been hard pressed to do without it.

Warning: Cactus plants are famous for their spines and the injuries they cause. But even more hazardous than the notorious spines are the glochids, the little barbed bristles, of which the *Opuntia* boasts many. These can cause extremely painful injuries. Handle this plant with the utmost care.

BIG ROOT

Marah fabaceus

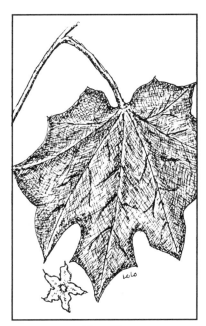

Big Root

Other names for the Big Root: Other popular names for this plant are Man Root, Wild Cucumber, and Suicide Plant. The Yuki Indians called it *Zhal-zhoi-e.* To the Calpella it was *Ma be-ha' yem*, to the Yokia, *He-te.*

Where to find it: Other species of this fascinating vine reside elsewhere in California, but *Marah fabaceus* generally grows only in Marin and Monterey counties, where it makes its home in scrubby places on banks and slopes and in mixed evergreen forests, seldom far from the coast. A variation of this species, however, *M. grestis* by name, thrives in other California counties including Mendocino, where it was used medicinally by several tribes of California Indians.

How to know it when you see it: This highly poisonous plant is a long and twining or high-climbing vine, characterized by an enormous fleshy root , often over a foot in diameter, the sight of which has historically sent imaginations soaring and blood running cold. Depending upon the eye of the beholder, it's the crouched figure of a human being, someone hunkered down, hiding in the earth like a mole; or it's a man's head, severed from the body, buried in the dirt by some heinous killer who still lurks in the forest, bent on foul play; or it's an ancient mummy, the gruesome remains of a monster dug up from its old-world grave and transplanted here in California.

The leaves of this oddity, three to six inches wide, are palmately lobed; its white flowers are flattish stars; its melons are spine-covered globes, filled with nut-like seeds that, apropos of its other grisly aspects, resemble those from which strychnine comes.

Its lore. Interestingly enough, according to oral history, either this plant's seeds, or the root for which it's named (or possibly both) were once used to put an end to human lives. Here, so it's said, was a suicide plant for Indians consumed by the death wish.

But Big Root was not only a killing plant; it was also a healing herb, and as such was greatly valued, prized especially as a treatment for such ailments as rheumatism and venereal disease. Sometimes the raw root was rubbed directly over the ailing parts. More often, however, it was roasted , a paste made of its ashes, and applied in a plaster or a poultice to the patient's flesh, there to remain until blisters formed as a certain sign that a cure was underway.

For other ills, especially urinary disorders, some Indians actually imbibed this dangerous poison—two charred seeds in the morning, and two in the evening, every day until the symptoms subsided.

Warning: Although Man Root is not listed in some books of poisonous plants, it is nonetheless reputed to be dangerously poisonous. Find it; eye it; enjoy its history. But otherwise leave it alone.

BLACKBERRY

Rubus spp.

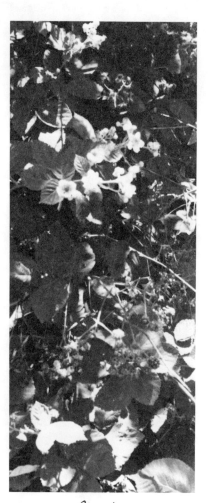

Blackberry

Other names for the Blackberry: Other common English names for this plant are California Blackberry, Common Blackberry, Brambles, and Bramble berry. The Yuki Indian name for the Blackberry was *Gol-le*. The Little Lake called it *T-ti-me*, while to the Concow it was *Wan-ko-mil-e*.

Where to find it: It could almost be said that blackberries and raspberries are found everywhere, for one or another of at least fifty species of this most beloved plant thrives in all fifty states.

How to know it when you see it: It's difficult to make a blanket description of the highly variable Blackberry bush, the bramble so beloved to herbalists, fruit lovers, pie bakers, and other inveterate berry pickers across the land. Some plants are thorny while others are not; some are showy while others are inconspicuous; some are only a few inches high while others rise up so tall that even on tiptoe the most diligent berry picker can't quite reach the luscious dark fruit at the top.

At least one favorite, the Cut-Leaf Blackberry, *Rubus laciniatus*, is happily easier to identify, for as its name implies, its leaves are keenly incised, and therefore distinguishable from those of its kin. This specimen is common by roadsides in damp places in the north of the state.

Its lore. Early visitors to California, men like Edwin Bryant, John Woodhouse Audubon, and Heinrich Lienhard, couldn't say enough about the delicious-looking fruit that met their eyes—and their bellies—while they were there. Bryant was a prominent journalist from Kentucky who traveled to California shortly before the gold rush and later wrote extensively of all that he saw there. Audubon was the son of the famous birder, himself a keen observer of the world of nature that his father loved so much. Lienhard was a Swiss immigrant, an avid diarist who first traveled to California in 1846, and penned lengthy descriptions of all he saw and did. All three of these sophisticated gentlemen saw fit to wax poetic about the berries.

Even though, according to his own testimony, Lienhard was so elated to be nearing the famous Sutter's Fort in the Sacramento Valley that he was shouting and throwing his hat in the air, he suspended such revelry long enough to stop and pick berries by the wayside. In his own words: "It was not long before the road swung toward the left and curved past a clump of willow on the bank of the American Fork where I saw some blackberry vines. Hungry for fresh fruit, I stopped long enough to pick a handful of these luscious berries. Unfortunately they stained my best suit, which I was wearing in honor of the occasion; it took me a long time and a considerable amount of scrubbing with cold water dipped out of the river to get it clean again. But the fruit was unbelievably delicious . . ."

Of course, long before Lienhard stained his suit there by the fork of the American River, blackberries were highly valued in that brambly wilderness called California. A favorite food of most all local Indians, sometimes eaten straight from the vine, sometimes dried and stashed away to serve as wintertime treats, this succulent fruit was also an indispensable medicine.

The berries and their juices, and sometimes an infusion of the salvific root, were long used by natives to treat stomach complaints, to lessen menstrual flow, to ease the wages of everyday stress, to allay vomiting , to prevent miscarriage, and to check diarrhea.

Indians and early settlers alike praised the blackberry as the best cure known for a case of indigestion. They found it powerful enough to soothe the belly rumblings of an overindulgent adult, yet mild enough for a colicky babe. For the infant, of course, a draught of plain juice was the common prescription, but for an ailing adult settler (even one who was generally a teetotaler) a jigger of blackberry brandy—as thick as syrup, as dark as burgundy wine—was often the order of the day.

Not just the berries themselves, but the roots and the leaves, were deemed remedial, too. A brew made from either leaf or root—as tasty, settlers claimed, as a cup of Chinese tea—was said to dry up runny noses, ease congestion, calm the nerves, and even serve as an antidote to certain poisons. As a gargle and mouth wash , an infusion of leaves or root was prescribed to dissolve tooth tartar, to heal canker sores, to cure bleeding gums, to treat coughs and scratchy throats, and do away with bad breath. When combined with honey and alum it was even reputed to tighten loose teeth.

In addition to all the above uses, blackberries, or their strained juices, were often added to other wild remedies, not only to render them more beneficial, but to make them more palatable as well. It's easy to see how, in one form or another, the beneficent blackberry used to find its way into every settler's larder, onto every table, into every woven basket, and into the berry-stained hands of all the little toddlers who ever wandered off into the bramble.

BLUE CURLS

Trichostema spp.

Other names for Blue Curls: Other names Californians have used for this plant are Woolly Blue Curls, Vinegar-Weed, Tarweed, Camphor Weed, and Turpentine Weed. The Wailaki Indians called it *Dots-chang-she-bog-i*. To the Yuki it was *Lel-mil*. To the Spanish Californios it was *Romero*.

Where to find it: The very common *T. lanceolatum* abounds over extensive areas of California and flourishes on dry plains and low hills, at altitudes usually below 2,600 feet. *T. lanatum* is at home on mountain slopes.

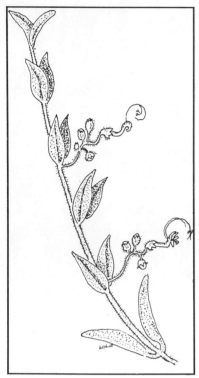

Blue Curls

How to know it when you see it: Blue Curls are strong-smelling members of the mint family, characterized by stiff stems, thin rosemary-like leaves, and odd-shaped, sometimes woolly, terminal flowers of pale purple or pink, which are arranged rather like those of some sage plants. *T. Lanceolatum*, often seen surrounded by the bees that love it, generally ranges in height from six to sixteen inches. *T. lanatum* is a leafy shrub that can reach heights of four feet, and is covered with a dense purple wool. A perfume to some nostrils, a stench to others, the strong scent of Blue Curls has been variously described as sagey, vinegar-like, camphor-smelling, and "turpentiney."

Its lore. The Cahuilla Indians used the leaves and the winsome flowers of *T. lanatum* to make a truly lovely-tasting and aromatic tea, which was said to be a good remedy for stomach troubles of literally every known variety. Another species of Blue Curls, *T. lanceolatum*—one that was also used by native anglers as a fish poison second only to Turkey Mullein—was considered medicinal by northern tribes such as the Concows, the Wailakis and the Yukis. An infusion of its leaves was an external wash for treating headaches, and, when combined with those of Turkey Mullein, a lotion applied to victims of typhoid. To the Chumash it was an even more important medicine, especially to mothers in labor; it was employed to help expel the placenta.

Today wild-food enthusiasts, survivalists, and herbal buffs alike are quick to extoll the virtues of Blue Curl Tea for its unique piney flavor, the wonderfully echoing aftertaste of its flowers, and its remarkable ability to settle upset stomachs.

BLUE GUM TREE

Eucalyptus Globulus

Other names for the Blue Gum Tree: Gum Tree, Eucalyptus Tree, Fever Tree. The Cahuilla Indians called this tree *Qahich'a waavu'it*.

Where to find it: As many as one hundred species of Australia's five hundred kinds of Eucalyptus trees are grown ornamentally in one place or another in the state of California and can be seen in yards, parks, and gardens here and there. But only three of these, *E. polyanthemos*, *E. Globulus*, and *E. tereticornis* have established themselves outside of cultivation and are growing wild. Generally when someone refers to a Eucalyptus tree, it's *E. Globulus*, the great Blue Gum tree, that they have in mind.

A very useful plant, which serves to dry out marshy areas where diseases might otherwise prevail—the Blue Gum tree favors locations where the average temperature ranges above 60°F.

How to know it when you see it: In California, the most typical Eucalyptus, *E. Globulus*, popularly known as Blue Gum, is an enormous evergreen that can reach three hundred feet. Its leaves (heart-shaped when young) are bluish-green, lance-shaped, smooth, and pungently aromatic. Its fruit is angular and equally aromatic. Its bark is quite beautiful, a smooth gray mottled with shades of pale pink, yellow, and blue.

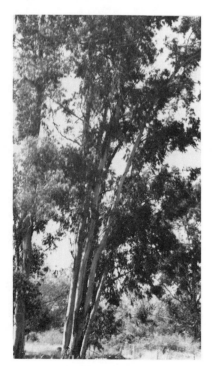

Blue Gum

Its lore. Although the Eucalyptus tree wasn't introduced into California until the nineteenth century, the desert Indians quickly discovered medicinal uses for this beautiful and useful alien from Tasmania. Cahuilla womenfolk, who found that its pollen made a fine facial cosmetic, knew how to concoct a Eucalyptus potion that served as a sedative for their wakeful or colicky infants. Other Californians, Indians and settlers alike, were also quick to take the plant to heart. It remains in favor today, a giant of a tree (one of the world's largest) cherished for its wood, its ornamental value, and its highly aromatic and antiseptic oil. A popular treatment for colds, coughs, bronchitis and asthma, it's an ingredient in ointments and salves, cough drops, syrups, and inhalants galore.

Caution: Some of the cultivated Eucalyptus trees, including the Manna Gum, *E. viminalis*; and the Sugar Gum, *E. cladocalyx*, are toxic enough to be lethal. The Sugar Gum, for example, is known to have caused the poisoning of livestock in its native land. The only toxic product of the giant Blue Gum tree, however, is its refined oil. If a human were to consume the oil (which is highly unlikely, except in case of accident or experimentation), he or she could suffer such symptoms as vomiting, confusion, vertigo, and coma. Occasionally the handling of the oil can cause blistering to the skin of some hypersensitive persons.

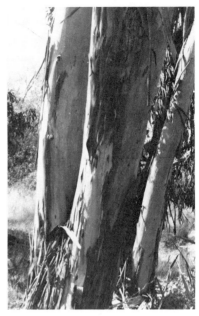

Blue Gum

BLUE VERVAIN

Verbena hastata

Other names for Blue Vervain: Other popular English names for this plant are Blue Verbena, Vervain, and Herb-of-the-Cross. To hispanic Californians this plant is *Moradilla*.

Where to find it: This fine medicinal plant is indigenous to the United States and found in moist places all over the American West. Swampy bottomlands are much to its liking.

How to know it when you see it: Growing sometimes as high as four feet tall, weed-like and hairy, Blue Vervain is a perennial herb with purplish flowers clustered at the end of an erect and slender spike. Its toothed leaves are opposite; its tiny seeds are best described as nutlets; in the right habitat it has the air of a weed and grows rampantly enough sometimes to be considered one.

Its lore. Though not quite so extravagant in their claims for this herb as Europeans in the middle ages, who thought it could ward away witchcraft, the first Californians held Blue Vervain in high esteem. The Concow Indians considered the root of the herb a superlative tonic, which they freely took for coughs and colds, or as a treatment for gout, or a soothing application for slow-healing wounds. Mixed with mistletoe and passionflower, it was supposedly an excellent tranquilizing tea, wonderfully calming to jangled nerves.

Early settlers agreed with the Concows; they already knew about Blue Vervain from the herbals they'd carried with them as they'd made the long trek

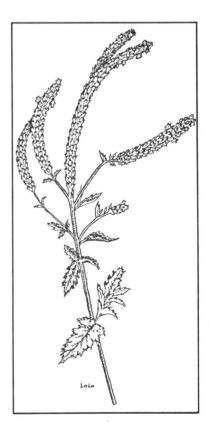

*Blue Vervain
(Western Verbena)*

westward, and were glad to find it growing in the California wilderness. Perhaps they even knew something of the legends that surrounded this much-revered wilding, such as the story that here was the plant that stanched the wounds of Christ on Calvary. Those who were religious may have taken this tale to heart, but chances are, most settlers who made use of Blue Vervain valued it most for its purported tranquilizing prowess, for which it's still praised today by many a modern herbalist.

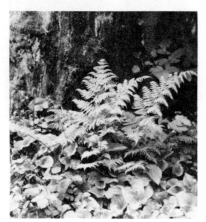

Bracken Fern

BRACKEN FERN

Pteridium aquilinum

Other names for Bracken Fern: Other popular English names for this plant are Bracken, Pasture Brake, Western Bracken, Brake Fern and Fiddlehead. The Calpella Indians called it *Bis*. To the Little Lake it was *Be-bi*; to the Concow, *S-la-la*; to the Numlaki, *Dos*. The Yokia called it *Ma-or-da-git*.

Where to find it: This hearty fern is so common it's sometimes looked upon with the sort of disdain that only an ugly weed should warrant. Unlike most ferns—shade dwellers and moisture lovers—Bracken abides in open, sunny places in woodlands, burns, and old pastures all across the country. In California it often shares habitat with plants such as Cow Parsnip, Golden Yarrow, and Pearly Everlasting.

How to know it when you see it: Look for a fern whose new fronds, which it keeps producing for months on end, are curled in such a way they resemble the tuning ends of violins. Aptly enough, these tender end parts are called "fiddleheads," and since they're entirely edible, wild-food enthusiasts are lately sampling such dishes as Bracken soup, or lettuce and Bracken salad, or even such gourmet dishes as Billy Joe Tatum's Bracken Fronds a l'Orange. All these, of course, are made of the young tender fiddleheads. Mature fronds are stiff and tough, dark green for the most part, but red-tinged at their bases, entirely unfit as food.

Its lore. Some California settlers, if they'd been schooled by Indians elsewhere on the continent, may have used a young-fiddlehead tea of tender-frond syrup to combat their own ills, especially liver complaints or lung disorders, which were said to respond well to such a decoction. If Delawares were among their teachers they might have used a Bracken rhizome tea to increase the flow of urine, while if their lessons came from the Ojibwa, they drank much the same brew for cramps.

Bracken was also considered powerful medicine for horses, and since Californians, especially the hard-riding Spaniards, were traditionally among the world's most avid horse fanciers, this meant that the plant was all the more prized.

Warning: Recent research shows that raw Bracken plants may be unsafe when consumed in large quantities. They contain an enzyme that can deplete the body of important vitamins. Other scientific tests indicate that overconsumption of Bracken Fern may lead to, or contribute toward, the development of stomach cancer.

BUFFALO GOURD

Cucurbita foetidissima

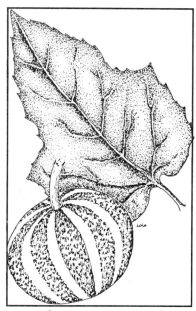

Buffalo Gourd

Other names for Buffalo Gourd: Another popular English name for this plant is Stinking Gourd. The Cahuilla Indians called it *Nekhish*. To California's hispanics it's *Calabasillo*.

Where to find it: Kin to the pumpkin, this trailing gourd plant is a denizen of many of California's sandiest, scrubbiest, and roughest places, especially in the southern parts of the state where it's equally at home on coastal strands, in sage scrub, on gravelly flats, in dry grasslands, or on the forbidding stretches of the Mojave Desert.

How to know it when you see it: A bold and brassy member of the cucumber family, blooming all through summer, this coarse perennial is better-known for its rank smell than for its big yellow male flower, a solitary bloom shaped like an up-turned bell, or even for the white-striped green gourds that quickly develop from the less showy female flowers. The root of the plant is enormous; its leaves are heart-shaped or triangular; its vines are long and trailing, sometimes growing up to 15 feet in length.

Its lore. Oldtimers used to mix the pulp of the Buffalo Gourd with soap and apply the resultant mass to sores and ulcers that other poultices and plasters had failed to cure. Or they'd liberally dust the suppurating parts with a quantity of pulverized dried seeds, which some averred was a far more healing application. Apparently, however, the root of the plant was its most beneficial part of all. Certainly it was the most versatile; with equal ease it could cure a bad case of piles or kill a mass of maggots infesting an open wound.

Cahuilla Indians used to chew the pulp of the Buffalo Gourd and apply the pithy mass to open sores, or boil the dried root and drink the decoction as either an emetic or a physic.

This herb was reputedly a fine horse medicine too. An unlikely mixture of crushed root and ordinary sugar was an old-standby poultice for the most stubborn saddle sores on horses.

CALIFORNIA BUCKEYE

Aesculus californica

Other names for the California Buckeye Tree: Other popular English names for this handsome tree are Buckeye, Fish Poison, Conquerors, Conkers, and Horse Chestnut. The Pomo Indian called it *De-sa Ka-la*, while the Yokia called it *Ba-sha*. To the Yuki it was *Sympt'ol*; to the Numlaki, *Far-sokt*.

Where to find it: The California Buckeye is a common tree in canyons and on dry slopes below 4,000 feet in many locations all through the state. Sometimes

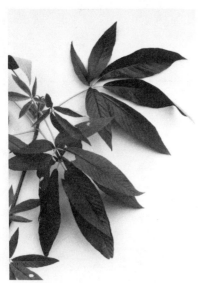

California Buckeye

it's found fraternizing with the typical trees of canyon floors: Big Leaf Maples, Willows, Cottonwoods, and Alders. But elsewhere, as on the hinterlands of the Great Central Valley, it's seen immixing with foothill plants like the Toyon and the Holly-leafed Cherry.

In Napa, Sonoma, and Mendocino counties this old-time medicinal seems to favor creekside banks where it's often surrounded by Blackberry bramble, Amole plants, and crimson tangles of Poison Oak.

How to know it when you see it: Smooth-barked, ranging in height from ten to forty feet, the California Buckeye is a small tree, sometimes quite scrubby-looking, but handsome nonetheless, especially in springtime and early summer when it's literally frosted all over with countless clusters of fragrant white or rose-colored flowers. In the fall, these showy panicles, five to ten inches long, are replaced by a wealth of luscious-looking fruit, which is clearly exposed when the leaves begin to fall just a month or two past flowering time.

The leaves of the Buckeye generally bear five leaflets each (though occasionally four or seven instead), which are oblong-lanceolate, four to six inches in length, and distinctly stemmed.

Its lore. The Pomo name for this native Californian, *De-sa ka-la*, translates into English as "fruit tree," which is precisely how these Indians perceived it: a producer and a yielder of a food they loved to eat. In a sense it's odd that they did, for the buckeye, unquestionably one of their favorite viands, wasn't even fit for consumption until after it had been pit-roasted for ten hours and leached for five days. Nonetheless this tree was prized first as a provider of food, only secondly as a remedy.

As to its purported medicinal properties, the Indians avowed that the buckeye fruit would expel bot worms from the bowels of their beloved horses, and that the bark of the tree would cure their own toothaches. Small fragments were placed in the cavity of the patient's offending tooth and kept firmly in place until, at last, the pain receded.

Warning: Raw California Buckeye fruit is deadly poisonous. One of several noted "suicide plants," Indians are said to have used it to take their own lives. The flowers, twigs, leaves and bark are also toxic. Human consumption may result in circulatory problems, restlessness, vomiting, involuntary elimination, diarrhea, twitching, poor coordination, dilated pupils, paralysis, and stupor. A few human fatalities have occurred in Europe due to consumption of toxic parts of *Aesculus* plants but there are none recorded in the United States.

The plant has caused abortion in cattle, and it's said that honeybees are sometimes poisoned by its pollen and nectar.

CALIFORNIA NUTMEG

Torreya californica

Other names for the California Nutmeg: Other English names are California Torreya and Torreya. To the Yokia Indians this tree was called *Ka-he*. To the Pomo is was *Ko-be* or *Ke-be*.

Where to find it: Look for the California Nutmeg tree on cool shaded slopes, in canyons, alongside streams, or in forests of mixed evergreens, Douglas Firs, or yellow pines.

How to know it when you see it: Growing thirty to ninety feet tall and resembling a young redwood tree , the California Nutmeg is a slender-branched evergreen with sharply-pointed leaves. Its fruit is variously described as "berry-like," "plum-like," "olive-like" and, ironically, much more rarely as "something like a nutmeg." Its bark is grayish-brown; its wood (a good candidate for fence posts), is as straw-hued as the coat of a yellow Labrador retriever.

Its lore. It was largely for the taste of its roasted fruit, said to be rather like that of peanuts, that this tree was so esteemed by the Indians. But it had other uses too, and these were not to be taken lightly. Its rigid leaves made excellent tattoo needles; its roots yielded a high-grade fiber for the exquisite baskets that the Pomo women wove. Furthermore, its strong, flexible, and spicy-tasting wood made excellent tools for dental hygiene, toothpicks of a sort, which were used to remove particles of food, clean the teeth, and help keep them healthy.

CALIFORNIA POPPY

Eschscholzia californica

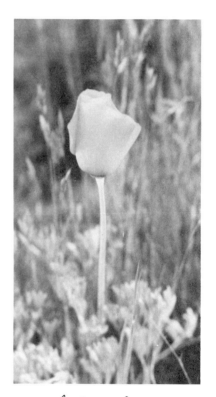

California Poppy

Other names for the California Poppy: The Yuki Indian name for the California Poppy was *Ho-yo-con-el*. The Little Lake called it *Ta-sha-le*, while to Wailaki it was *Tso-ta-ta-sit-cho*, and to the Cahuilla, *Tesinat*. To the Spanish Californios it was *Dormidera*, "the drowsy one," and *Copa de oro*, "cup of gold."

Where to find it: This bright-visaged plant, the state flower of California, is a common sight in an assortment of open places that run the gamut from grasslands to city parks, from cool Pacific slopes to the parched desert lands of the wide Mojave.

How to know it when you see it: Look for lacy green leaves that bear a vaguely bluish cast, and a four-petaled, bowl-shaped flower that may range in color from the fieriest orange to a pale creamy yellow.

Its lore. In another era, when the Spanish explorers first came to California, the hillsides in the coastlands were so poppy-bedecked and so breathtakingly bright that they named that region the Land of Fire.

Latter-day adventurers were equally captivated by this colorific native. A miner by the name of Peter Decker, who traveled overland to California in 1849, even wrote about the poppies in his diary. It's true they weren't the gold he'd come seeking, but they were golden nonetheless and he couldn't help but describe how they studded the hills near a place called Park's Bar.

Long before the miners came bustling, and even before the Spaniards came riding over the hills, the native California Indians were "mining" these poppies for all they were worth. They were busy decocting their salves, their teas and tonics, their tisanes and syrups, one or more of which, they must have reasoned, would surely cure whatever ailment might come along to plague them. In one of these forms or another they used the poppy to treat toothaches, insomnia, headaches, infected sores, slow-healing ulcers, unresponsive lovers, nervousness and stress, vomiting attacks, stomach-aches, and consumption. Some of the desert tribes even used this plant as a sedative to calm their fussing infants.

Warning: Every part of the California Poppy is toxic. The plant is slightly narcotic and has a depressant effect upon breathing.

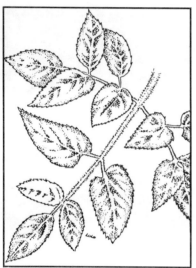

California Spikenard

CALIFORNIA SPIKENARD

Aralia californica

Other names for the California Spikenard: Other English names for this plant are California Ginseng and Spikenard. The Pomo Indians called it *Gos-e-zi so*, which translates as "elk clover." To the Yuki it was *Bu-ki-muk*, to the Concow, *Mal-e-me*.

Where to find it: This towering herb resides in moist and shady places from Orange County northward all the way to Oregon. You'll find it in deep canyons, and by the sides of creeks and running brooks. Look for it it too in deep Redwood groves where you're apt to find it mingling with Poison Oak, Salal, Oregon Grape, and other berries.

How to know it when you see it: Growing sometimes to heights of nine or ten feet, bearing ball-like umbels atop its huge fleshy stems, this towering member of the Ginseng family looks like a giant stalk of celery transplanted from some outlandish dreamscape.

Its lore. The aromatic roots of this giant herb were of such value that some Indians traveled miles to find it, and then thereafter kept in in their households where they showed it off to visitors with certain pride. It was a valuable commodity. Once dried, it was made into a decoction that—although reputedly good medicine for minor ailments like the common cold—was apparently generally reserved for the treatment of serious maladies like diseases of the lungs and stomach that might not respond to potions less powerful.

CANCHALAGUA

Centaurium venustum

Other names for the Canchalagua: Other popular English names for this plant are California Centaury and Charming Centaury. The Luiseno Indians used to call it *Ashoshkit*.

Where to find it: Canchalagua is a plant that seeks dry slopes and flats, chaparral country, coast sage scrub, and even desert edges, from Plumas County southward; common in and near Yosemite Valley, but more abundant the further south you go.

How to know it when you see it: Low to the earth (seldom over a foot high, often considerably shorter), not particularly noteworthy before it's bloomed, Canchalagua is best identified by its lovely flowers that grace their various habitats from May to August. Five-petaled, shaped like flat stars, they're reminiscent of pinwheels—those bits of folded plastic tacked to wooden dowels—that today's children carry about at carnivals, holding them up to the breeze as they run. Of course Canchalagua flowers don't whirl, but they're colorful (rose-colored, white, or yellow-throated) and they lend a festive air to the dry habitats where they thrive.

Its lore. Unmentioned in modern herbals, Canchalagua was once the talk of California, an old stand-by cure-all to the Indians, the prized panacea of every Spaniard's household, often found hanging in bunches from the hacienda rafters. Here was a commodity in great demand, often coveted, always sought, sometimes traded—even begged for and sent all the way to the Polynesian Islands, where it was eagerly awaited by Spaniards and Americans living in that distant land.

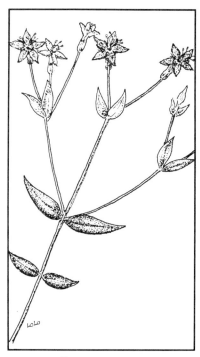

Canchalagua

If Canchalagua was second to any other medicinal herb in California then it could only have been to Angelica, and only then because the latter was so inextricably tied to the worship of the Indians who used it that its religious/spiritual connotations lent it extraordinary virtue. At any rate, there's ample testimony to the fact that *Centaurium venustum* was once widely extolled for virtues far beyond the beauty of its flowers.

In a letter he wrote to a friend in 1828, the prominent Californio herb enthusiast Jose M. de Estudillo had this to say of Canchalagua: ". . . I suppose that you already know of its great virtues, principally to reduce fevers, dropsy, kidney stones in the urine, and that it should not be taken very frequently together, and if at all, only two or three times a month, at three separate times. I experimented with it for six consecutive months by taking it every three days in the following manner:

"An infusion of three separate leaves was placed in a glass of water, more than one-fourth full, at five o'clock in the afternoon. The following day in the morning I took it and went for a walk. It relaxed my stomach and I urinated with a great deal of ease. With what it achieved, the bloated abdomen which suffocated me when walking went down, and it thinned the blood which I needed to have done so that I find myself agile today."

Americans like Alfred Robinson, a young clerk from Boston who came to California years before the gold rush, were equally enthusiastic in what they had to say about Canchalagua. According to him, it was "found to be excellent in curing the fever and ague, and may be depended upon in any case, no matter of how long standing. It abounds all over the coast, and in the spring, during the season of flowers, its pretty blossoms add much to the beauty of the country."

Another American, the accomplished journalist Edwin Bryant, also expounded on the virtues of this one-time king of California cure-alls. According to him, it was held by the Californians as "an antidote for all the diseases to which they are subject, but in particular for cases of fever and ague. For purifying the blood, and regulating the system, I think it surpasses all the medicinal herbs that have been brought into notice and must become in time, one of the most important articles in the practice of medicine. In the season for flowers, which is generally during the months of May and June, its pretty pink-colored blossoms form a conspicuous display in the great variety which adorn the fields of California."

CASCARA BUCKTHORN

Rhamnus purshiana

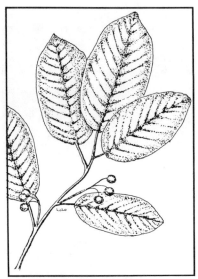

Cascara Buckthorn

Other names for the Cascara Buckthorn: Other English names for this plant are Cascara Sagrada, Sacred Bark, Chittem Bark, and Persian Bark. The Yokia Indian name for this tree was *Ho-sa ka-la*. To the Yuki it was *Um-pe* or *Tun-ti*, to the Concow, *Po*, and to the Wailaki *Sast-ket-a*.

Where to find it: Native to the Pacific Northwest, Cascara Buckthorn is most at home in forested locations, on mountain slopes, in canyons, and bottomlands, from British Columbia to Northern California.

How to know it when you see it: Look for a small deciduous tree, with finely-toothed alternate leaves that are vibrant green, that are roundish at the base, but can be either blunt or sharp at their ends. In spring you'll find this native northwesterner bearing little clusters of whitish-green flowers that will later develop into the cascara fruit, small black globes, each containing two or three seeds. This is an unobtrusive tree, seldom over thirty feet tall, with a trunk that averages only one and a half feet in diameter. There's nothing spectacular about its appearance, nothing whatever to tell you how useful it is and what a colorful history it boasts.

Its lore. When the Spanish padres first came to this new land they were just as alert to the healing arts of the Indians here as their countrymen had been to those of the natives of Mexico, from whom they'd learned enough to fill volumes. It was little wonder that they were so attentive, for mission priests were often called upon to treat the ills of their parishioners, Indian and fellow Spaniard alike. In fact, sometimes these overworked friars were looked upon as doctors, while the missions they administrated were thought of as infirmaries. (At least one such establishment, Mission San Rafael in northern California, was actually founded for the purpose of hospitalizing ailing Indians.) It was truly of vital importance that they should learn all they could about native medicinal plants, where they were found, how they were used, and what cures they wrought. Later, if a particular plant was proven effective, they'd use it themselves; they'd prescribe it for their ailing flock; they'd write about it in letters to relatives and friends or fellow priests in Mexico or Spain. They'd barter with it, trading this herb for that, favor for favor, cure for cure. So it was with the wonderful Cascara Buckthorn tree, which they called by a name that the Indians too began to use: Cascara Sagrada, the "sacred bark."

Some individuals, especially those who've never suffered irregularity, may argue that a treatment for constipation (the prime usage of this old medicinal plant) scarcely deserves the label "sacred." But blessed or not, one thing is certain: Cascara works. In fact, it works so well that, unlike most old folk remedies, it's still popular today after many long decades of constant use.

CASTOR BEAN

Ricinus communis

Other names for the Castor Bean: To the Cahuilla Indians this plant was *Navish*. The early Spanish Californios called it *Palma Christi*.

Where to find it: This lethal member of the Spurge family, a native of Asia, sometimes cultivated for ornamental purposes, is found growing wild in waste places and in sage scrub country along the coast.

How to know it when you see it: The leaves of this alien shrub are palmately five-lobed, dark green in color and, when full size, measure as much as two and a half feet in width. Its flowers are pinkish, its fruit spiny, and its rather attractive, smooth, glossy seeds are speckled and mottled like a songbird's eggs. The plant grows from 3 to 10 feet high.

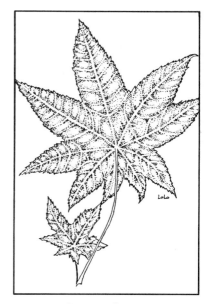

Castor Bean

Its lore. The famous old medicament, that king among cathartics best known as castor oil, is derived from the pretty speckled seeds of this plant. Be it known, however, that the process by which the effective oil is extricated from the seeds is a complex one and in no way the province of the folk-medicine enthusiast. This is a very poisonous plant. It's so dangerous, in fact, that adults who share its habitat are constantly warning their children to avoid it. The author recollects, with a shudder, a time when one of her own toddlers failed to heed her words of admonition. She found him just as he was ready to bite into a Castor Bean, which he'd peeled and poked in his mouth, because the white pithy substance looked to him, so he said, "just like popcorn, Mommie." If she hadn't discovered him in the act, he might not have lived to share in the telling of the story.

As was the case with many a poisonous plant, however, the Indians put the Castor Bean to use medicinally. When the pernicious seeds were ripe, some of the desert tribes peeled and mashed them and applied the greasy yield—as a salve or pack or plaster—to their sores, to soothe them and help them to heal.

One of the best-known and most-used store-bought medicaments of the late nineteenth and early twentieth centuries, commercially extracted castor oil is still a favorite remedy of many California residents, especially old-timers like Sonoma County's well known writer and horsewoman, Natlee Kenoyer. Prized recruit of the National Cowgirl Hall of Fame, still writing western stories and teaching horsemanship although she's over eighty, Natlee touts castor oil as a soothing external rub for the occasional aches and pains that have yet to keep her off a horse's back.

Warning: As they contain Ricin, one of the most dangerous substances known, the seeds, and to a lesser extent the leaves, of the castor oil plants are extremely toxic. The Ricin is released into the mouth of the victim when the seeds (as few as two of which can prove fatal to a child) are broken and chewed.

CATTAIL

Typha latifolia

Other names for the Cattail: Other common English names for this plant are Rushes, Flags, Bulrush, Cat-o-Nine Tails, and Soft Flag. The Cahuilla name for the plant was *Ku'ut*.

Where to find it: A proliferate wilding, the Cattail thrives in ponds and swamps, in marshes, by lakes, near streams, or in any other marshy fresh-water habitat throughout the west. In this case, "marshy habitats" can be said to include even gullies, ditches, and other damp declivities within the confines of certain city limits. Take the North Bay town of Santa Rosa, for example, where it grows on the grounds of an outskirt shopping center—"The Crossroads," by name—in a would-be marsh only a few yards long, situated behind a small florist's shop where shoppers coming and going seem not to notice it bowing gracefully in the wind.

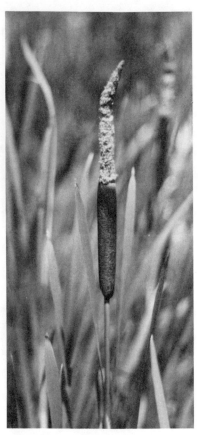

Cattail

How to know it when you see it: There are few medicinal plants in the world easier to identify than the almost-ubiquitous, once marvelously useful Cattail. As its popular name implies, its most conspicuous feature is its "tail," which is really nothing more (and nothing less) than its countless flowers, densely packed in a cylindrical brown spike at the end of a long stout stalk.

Other than the tail, *Typha latifolia's* distinguishing features are its long, tapering leaves, which move in the breeze like starched sashes on a clothesline.

Its lore. Early settlers and California Indians had so many uses for these tall graceful plants that the list, running the gamut from food to folk medicine, is practically endless. The highly edible and nutritious young shoots and the pollen were consumed both raw and cooked. The starchy roots were generally roasted or boiled, except when they were dried and ground into flour. Even the leaves, though rarely eaten, didn't go to waste. These served to caulk barrels, to make rush-bottom furniture, to fashion rugs and mats and shades.

As to its medicinal uses, the Cattail shone here too. While the roots of the plant were enlisted to heal open wounds, stem preparations were taken internally to cure diarrhea, to kill worms, and to treat venereal disease. Similar concoctions served as external applications for cuts, burns and stubborn sores. But it was the contents of the tail itself, the wondrous Cattail "down," soft as goose feathers, that was the greatest boon to the innovative residents of early California. Here was a peerless dressing for sores and lacerations, a soothing covering for diaper rashes and seven-year itches, soft bedding for an ailing child or a mother giving birth.

Cattail hasn't lost its usefulness. In recent times, it's been used as a filling for life jackets, as a soundproofing material, and as insulation for walls and ceilings. But whatever its uses now or in the future, it's doubtful it'll ever be prized as highly as it was in the days when one could eat Cattail-flour bread at a table set with Cattail-rush mats, or sit on a Cattail-down pillow in a Cattail-rush-bottomed rocking chair, rocking a baby whose poor sore posterior had just been soothed with a soft dossil of Cattail down.

CENTURY PLANT

Agave deserti

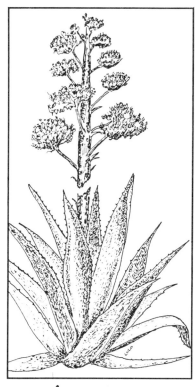

Century Plant

Other names for the Century Plant: To the early Spanish Californios this plant was known as *Mescal*.

Where to find it: *Agave deserti*, best known as the Century Plant, is one of several *Agaves* found growing in dry regions of the great southwest, in both the high and low deserts, in dry ground, on slopes, and in washes at altitudes that generally range from 1,500 to 5,000 feet.

How to know it when you see it: When it's in bloom, which, according to legend occurs only once in a century, in the month of May, there's probably no plant on the face of the earth easier to identify than this useful old denizen of the California deserts. Its hefty stalk rises up like a flag pole and scrapes the sky with its yellow flowers. These sunny blooms appear in clumps like separate bouquets arranged by a shaman who means to share them with the watchful gods. Beneath these flowers, at the base of the stalk, is a whorl of spiky leaves, sharp-tipped, sharp-edged, and lethal-looking, which is all there is to see of the Century Plant during those many long years (actually considerably less than a century) when it's not in bloom.

It's an interesting fact that once the fruit of the *Agave deserti* has matured, it's time for the rest of the plant to die.

Its lore. A Desert Agave in bloom is a captivating sight, even to those who have no idea what a historic event they're witnessing. To a desert dweller who's heard and believed the legend of the Century Plant and then finds one blooming in her own back yard, it's nothing short of awe-inspiring. Eighty-five year old Viola Vallier, a long-time resident of Palm Springs, still talks about the time one bloomed by her door the year that she was 50. "I just kept thinking how long it had taken for it to sprout those flowers," she says, shaking her head, "and how old it was. And what stories it would have to tell me if it could only talk."

If the Century Plant *could* talk it would doubtless tell about the days when it was a storehouse of food and beverages and weaving fiber for a grateful lot of Indians and settlers who counted it amongst the blessings that the desert vouchsafed them. It might tell too how the natives once used its potent juices as a diuretic, and how sometimes, hopefully, though not quite so successfully, they used it too as an antisyphilitic, which they sorely needed after the coming of the white man.

Warning: Among the many individuals who have suffered severely from trying to uproot or chop down a plant of this genus, and who can testify, therefore, that contact with some species of *Agave* can cause a "violent and frenzied itching," are two Sonoma County residents, Jim Westrich and Michael Sims. In 1987 these gentlemen took a chain saw to a particular backyard plant that was proving to be a menace to children at play. They were so badly afflicted after only a few moments of contact that they rushed frantically into the house, peeled off their clothing immediately, took long showers, and dabbed themselves liberally with an assortment of itch medications. According to their description, they were almost "crazy with discomfort." As extreme as these symptoms were, however, no permanent damage was done. Within an hour the violent itching had subsided completely.

CHICORY

Chichorium intybus

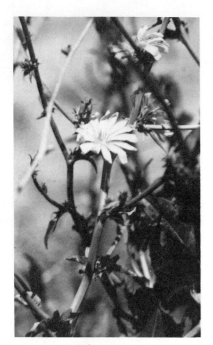

Chicory

Other names for Chicory: Other popular English names for this plant are Blue Dandelion, Blue Daisy, Blue Sailors, Ragged Sailors, Blowball, Succory, Wild Endive, and Wild Bachelor Button.

Where to find it: This useful Eurasian is naturalized over most of the United States. In California it escaped from commercial cultivation in Steinbeck's beloved Salinas Valley and is now found growing along roadsides, in untended yards, vacant lots, and open fields, especially in Monterey and Sonoma Counties.

How to know it when you see it: Chicory is best known for its prominent daisy-like flowers which, though occasionally pale pink or off white, are usually a vibrant shade of blue, vaguely tinged with violet, and so lovely to look at they defy description. On sunny days their petals close at noontime, at which time the plant becomes a homely weed, not one whit more attractive than the dandelion it resembles. But sometimes when the sun stays hidden, the blooms remain open all day, colorful and showy, and as pleasing to the eye as any garden flower.

Its lore. Chicory played no role in the folk medicine of the California Indians or the early Hispanic residents. It wasn't a native plant; it was never a favorite of the Spaniards. Apparently it wasn't even cultivated in the mission padres' famous gardens, where according to frequent testimony, you could expect to find almost any useful plant suitable to the habitat. And yet to the latter-day settlers who came to California after the gold rush, many of them carrying seeds of their choice herbs in their pockets or in their packs, Chicory (which, incidentally, is easily grown from seed) was worthwhile indeed. If they were amongst those who still clung to the age-old belief in the Doctrine of Signatures, they probably believed that, because of its milk-like sap, it was an excellent herb for nursing mothers. They almost surely used it as a laxative, as a diuretic, as a general tonic, and as the makings of poultices for swellings and inflammations, rashes and sores.

Chicory is rarely used medicinally nowadays. Still, it's not forgotten; it's a coffee additive or substitute; it's a salad green; it's a seasoning for stews. But best of all, perhaps, when its blue flowers are blooming it's a volunteer beautifier of homely waste places in those California counties where it's taken root.

CLOVER

Trifolium spp.

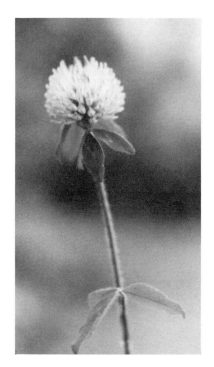

Clover

Other names for Clover: The Pomo Indian name, *So*, signified not only all Clover plants in general but also other plants that were eaten green and in the uncooked state. The Cahuilla name for Clover in general was *Tre'evula*. To the early Spanish Californios Clover was *Trebol*.

Where to find it: With flower heads that vary from the deepest crimson to purest of whites, many species of Clover flourish in the California soil. Some are native to the land; some are aliens from Europe. Look for Clover in meadows and pastures, in city parks and backyards, along roadsides, and in open woods.

How to know it when you see it: Like the dandelion, Clover is such a familiar sight that it's usually easily identified even by those to whom "the great outdoors" is nothing more than the local city park. This is so true that a description seems almost superfluous. Suffice it to say the California Clovers are all common weeds, members of the pea family, and that they bear heads of densely-compacted little pea-like flowers, and leaflets that generally come in threes.

The hairy-stemmed Red Clover, an alien well-established in America, bears pinkish flowerheads and green leaves, each of which is marked with the shape of a V. It grows in clumps up to heights of nearly three feet.

Its lore. To the Indians of California, Clover was more than a familiar weed. Like the acorn, it was not only a part of their diet, but a vital part of their lives. Inextricably woven into the warp threads of their psyches, its significance was such that it affected them physically, socially, and spiritually. This kind of overlapping from one of life's aspects to another was natural to the Indian. It was not his nature to compartmentalize; he didn't live in an "either/or" world. If you'd asked a Yoki or a Wailaki if Clover was a food or a medicine, he'd have found the question foolish. Clover was a seasonal treat, the consumption of which was almost a purification rite; it was a spring tonic; its harvest was cause for fellowship. It was a nutritious health-fortifying gift of the Earth for which to give thanks; it was an inspiration, a reason for contemplation and prayer. It was cause too for revelry; there were Clover dances to celebrate its ripening; there were Clover games to play and chants to chant.

Although the flowers of several species were also relished, as was the seed of a few, it was the green foliage, fresh and sweet and tender, picked before the flowers bloomed, that was most favored by the natives. Right up until the beginning of the twentieth century, it was a common and colorful sight in spring and early summer to see small groups of Indians stepping out of the lush fields and meadows carrying the sweet crisp stems of this much-favored food tied in their big red bandanas.

Settlers used to wonder how the Indians managed to eat with impunity a food that was known to cause bloating in cattle. It's possible (as V. K. Chestnut conjectured in a book he wrote about plant uses of the Round Valley Indians of the late 1800s) that the natives made a point of accompanying a meal of Clover with some substance they knew would counteract its potential ill effects—Peppernut, for example. Nonetheless, sometimes the Indians, too, paid for their feasting with distended bellies. The Patwins of the San Francisco Bay region even had a prescription for the treatment of Clover bloat: a quantity of the extract of Amole rubbed externally on the ailing stomach until its discomforts were eased. Nutritious and protein-rich as it is, there's no question about it: raw Clover is hard to digest. In fact, most modern-day wild-food enthusiasts suggest that it be soaked in salt-water or cooked before it's eaten.

Although a few settlers occasionally used Clover as a food themselves, others shuddered at the idea that human beings would eat a plant that, according to their perceptions, was quite plainly intended only as fodder for the beasts of the fields. To their way of thinking, it was one thing to use the plant as a medicinal herb (as many of them did), but to use it as food was another matter entirely, and one they saw as so unsavory that they were suspect of anyone who didn't feel the same as they did. Hence, some less provincial souls, like the illustrious Captain John August Sutter, the so-called "Father of California," were often accused of *compelling* the natives to forage for their food. According to amateur ethnologist Stephen Powers, who visited California in 1871 and 1872, this was hardly the case. As he saw it, "Captain Sutter's Indians preferred to eat clover for a change and a relish, and he simply--let them do it."

Doubtless, even some of those settlers who turned up their noses at Clover as a food were only too happy to use the plant medicinally. This was especially true of European immigrants, many of whom had the highest esteem for their own *Trifolium pratense*, best known as Red Clover, that had happily become naturalized in California. At least a pinch of their loyalty to this old folk remedy may have been based on age-old superstitions that hailed from England, where the leaves of the plant were once worn as a charm against witches, or from Ireland, where another species of *Trifolium*, the legendary shamrock, had for centuries been synonymous with good luck. But superstitious or not, these settlers firmly believed in the healing prowess of Clover. Hadn't their own sore throats improved when they'd taken doses of Clover syrup? Hadn't that same medicament eased their youngsters' whooping cough? Weren't the news articles of the day extolling the benefits of Red Clover tea to victims of cancer?

Although modern pharmacologists find no scientific data to validate the medical uses of this old-favorite herb, many herbalists still tout its use as an alterative and as an aid to general health; many a health-food advocate avidly drinks her morning cup of Clover tea; and the number of wild-food enthusiasts who are cooking up a quantity of the Indian's old-favorite food "for a change and a relish" appears to be steadily growing.

Warning: Never eat uncooked Clover. It's extremely hard to digest. According to experts the entire plant is toxic. Symptoms of poisoning in animals are infertility and an effect on the rate of growth.

COAST ERIOGONUM

Eriogonum latifolium

Other names for the Coast Eriogonum: The Yuki Indians called this plant *Al-bo-te*.

Where to find it: You'll find this interesting and widespread member of the Buckwheat family in sandy places on coastline cliffs from central California to Oregon.

How to know it when you see it: The leaves of the Coast Eriogonum, which are clustered densely together at the base of their stout stems, are oblong, wavy-margined, and woolly on their undersides. The stems themselves are entirely leafless, sometimes wand-like but more often branching out in such a way as to look unkempt, and bearing at their ends a number of white or rose-colored flowers, which look like small round balls skewered on forked sticks.

Its lore. Coast Eriogonum may be something less than beautiful, yet there was a time when this unprepossessing plant was sought after with considerable zeal. In the spring of the year—before the days when radio and television kept them transfixed indoors—the children of California used to run about the hillsides seeking their beloved "sour grass," breaking off the tender young stems to suck and savor.

   Adults had other reasons to clamour for the Coast Eriogonum, for here was a plant that ranked high on their compendium of California cures. From its woody root, so potent it could be used over and over, they decocted remedies for ailments such as headaches, stomach-aches, sore eyes, and that long and colorful string of maladies termed under the general heading of "female complaints."

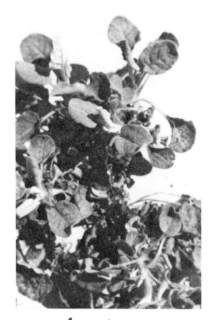

Coast Eriogonum before blooming

COFFEEBERRY

Rhamnus californica

Other names for the Coffeeberry Tree: Another common name for this tree is California Buckthorn. The Cahuilla Indians used to call it *Hoon-wet-que-wa* or *Hun qwa'i'va'a*, which means "what the bear eats."

Where to find it: Coffeeberry favors rocky hillsides, beach dunes, chaparral country, shaded slopes, and assorted ravines and arroyos at altitudes below 3,500 feet. You may find it growing near the big gnarled fire pines in the shadows of groves that seem ghost-haunted and eerie, or in the company of coast live oaks in woodlands that are park-like and more serene.

How to know it when you see it: Sometimes a small tree, twenty feet tall, upright and rounded, sometimes a low and spreading four-foot shrub, Coffeeberry has reddish twigs, narrowly elliptical leaves, small flowers of green, and fruit that's black and berry-like.

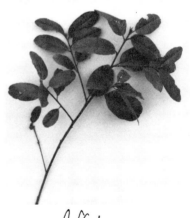

Coffeeberry

Its lore. Like its relative the Cascara Buckthorn, this native plant was considered by the Indians and the Spaniards, and other early settlers as well, to be almost sacred, and the cures it wrought nothing short of wondrous. The usual method of preparation was a simple one: a handful of bark in a gallon of ordinary drinking water, boiled until the mixture "tasted like wine." A simple decoction, to be sure, but one reputed to cure ailments much more complex than the common constipation for which it was so often used. In the late 1800s, Round Valley residents claimed that three cups of this potion cured a man who was suffering so severely from what they referred to as "mania," that they'd had to keep him in restraints.

For ailments less severe, or simply as a tonic to improve the appetite or restore general health, some settlers used to soak the dried bark of the Coffeeberry overnight in a glass of water and then drink that bracing brew first thing in the morning.

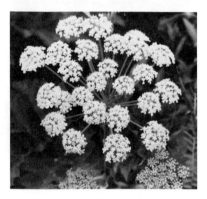

Cow Parsnip

COW PARSNIP

Heracleum lanatum

Other names for the Cow Parsnip: This plant is also sometimes called Cow Cabbage and Masterwort. To the Yuki Indians it was *Mun-shok*. The Yokia called it *Ta-ra-tit*, whereas its Concow name was *Chou-me-o*. The Spanish name for Cow Parsnip is *Concha*.

Where to find it: This oversized member of the carrot family dwells on sea cliffs from Monterey County to Alaska, in the mountains below 9,000 feet, and in moist thickets and other shaded places where it's sometimes found keeping company with plants such as Sword Fern, Paintbrush, and Blue Blossom Ceanothus. In the springtime, when it's in full bloom, there's no more familiar sight in certain northern California locations like Mendocino and Sonoma Counties than this giant perennial.

How to know it when you see it: Reaching sometimes to a height of eight feet, the hollow-stemmed Cow Parsnip is a towering plant, an imposing, if somewhat homely, sight to behold when it's in full bloom. Tall and erect, it bears great flat umbels of white flowers, "flapjack faces, upturned to the sun," as one California poet so aptly described them, and big, lobed, green leaves that measure up to twenty inches wide.

Its lore. Records indicate that California Indians valued Cow Parsnip most especially as a food. In the spring of the year, before its flowers had developed, they found its tender leaves and flower stalks as sweet-tasting as they were aromatic. But *Heracleum lanatum* did have its role to play in regional folk medicine too. It's said that in the days before the gold rush, the early Spanish residents of California used a strong decoction of its roots as an external treatment for rheumatism. Its possible that they learned of this remedy from the Indians themselves, for however much the natives favored it as a food, they could not have failed to discover other uses for this towering plant. Was it they or the

Spaniards who taught latter-day settlers of its other medicinal uses? Or did those frontier folk bring their recipes for Cow Parsnip decoctions with them when they made the long trek westward? One way or the other, at one time or another, down through the decades, California's wild-plant enthusiasts have used this stout old perennial as a remedy for intestinal disorders, headaches, indigestion, gas, cramps, and even epilepsy.

Warning: Cow Parsnip shares habitats with several poisonous plants whose descriptions are similar. If in doubt, don't even touch the plant in question.

CREEPING JENNY

Convolvulus arvensis

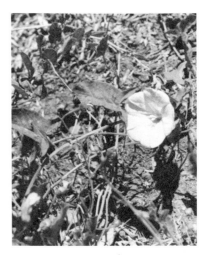

Creeping Jenny

Other names for Creeping Jenny: This common weed is also known as Field Bindweed, Wild Morning Glory, Small-flowered Morning Glory, Corn Lily, Lap-love, Sheep-bine, Corn-bind, and Bear Bind.

Where to find it: Creeping Jenny makes its home in disturbed places all up and down the Pacific states, on roadsides and footpaths, in fields and orchards, lawns and gardens, and vacant lots.

How to know it when you see it: With its pointed lobes, the mat-green leaves of this twining and much-detested weed are shaped much like the spades that are so often used to dig it up from the garden and cast it with a vengence into the trash bin. Its trumpet-shaped flowers, whose undeniable beauty seems almost a mockery to the gardeners and farmers it plagues, are a distinct rose-color before they open, a papery white thereafter, just barely tinged with the palest of pinks.

Deep-rooted and persistent, wherever Creeping Jenny grows it grows in wild profusion. The fields or roadsides where you find it are so full of it they're like bolts of polka-dot fabric, rolled out and ready for the dressmaker's scissors. Sometimes these same plots of ground are home to Chicory plants—in which case vibrant blue and rose-washed white complement each other so well that even the most zealous weed exterminator, armed with his hoe or his sodium chlorate, cannot deny that here indeed is a lovely sight.

In a word, you can't miss Creeping Jenny, even if you want to.

Its lore. This hearty little bindweed is such a well-established and common resident of California, it's hard to believe that it's really an alien, that it hails from Eurasia, that there was once a day when it wasn't here at all. But it's true, Creeping Jenny is not a native plant, it was never a prized herb of the Indians, the Spaniards never cultivated it in their gardens, no thanks-giving ceremony was given it its honor, no chants sung in its praise. It *is* a Californian now, however, and it is an age-old remedy, and as such, it does rate mention in a compendium of California folk medicine. Although it has never been used as much as its relative, the showier Hedge Bindweed, its properties are much the same. This is true of all the bindweeds from the the crimson-flowered Jalap of Mexico to the Syrian plant called Scammony. Bindweed has been used as a laxative, as a treatment for jaundice, and as a remedy for gall-bladder problems.

CREOSOTE BUSH

Larrea divaricata

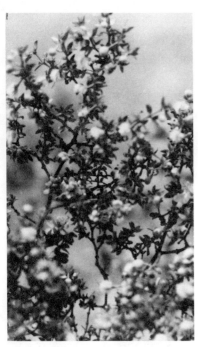

Creosote Bush

Other names for the Creosote Bush: Two other popular English names for this plant are Greasewood and Chaparral. To California's hispanic population it is *Hediondilla*. The Cahuilla Indians used to call it *Atukul*.

Where to find it: Typical of the Colorado and Mojave Deserts, sometimes surviving long periods without rainfall, this native scrub is at home in gullies and washes and sage brush plains as surely as it is in the more hospitable desert oases. There's no more adaptable plant in all of the West. In fact, although it's sometimes found surrounded by other desert dwellers like Buckwheat, Mormon Tea, Bladder Sage, Desert Trumpet, and Indigo Bush, there are many areas in the desert where it's the only vegetation to be seen for miles. Sometimes this plant is grown in gardens of native plants, where, surprisingly enough, it's considered ornamental.

How to know it when you see it: A many-branched resinous evergreen, rarely growing over nine feet tall, the Creosote Bush bears olive-green leaves that grow in opposite pairs, each one consisting of two tiny leaflets that are thick, shiny, and sometimes sticky to the touch. Its flowers, which are five-petaled and yellow, appear in spring and are followed in early summer by its fruit, showy white seed balls covered with fuzz.

Its lore. High-school girls sauntering across washes on the outskirts of old Palm Springs used to break off twigs of this plant and place them in their billfolds next to their identification cards. It appealed to that keen teen-age sense of drama to think that, in case of accident, whoever found them would read their wordless message, "I love the desert," loud and clear. Besides, when they opened up their purses the resinous scent of Creosote wafted up to meet their noses and remind them that they'd sealed themselves forever to the winds and sands of home.

Melodramatic though it was, the behavior of these youngsters was not far out of character for desert-bred Californians. To many people who live in arid spots like that old haunt of the Agua Caliente Indians, the Creosote bush is as sweet a sight and as sure a sign of home as any hearth or rocking chair or rose bush in the garden. And that pungent odor (the same that rose up from the students' pocketbooks), especially strong when the rains come and the leathery leaves grow sticky, is as welcome to the nostrils of the true "desert rat" as the scent of tarred wharf pilings to a fisherman.

Comparisons like these are effective as far as they go, but since it can scarcely be said that rocking chairs and old pilings are prized for their medicinal properties, they don't go far enough. They've nothing to say for the role of this remarkable plant in the folk medicine of its people, especially those herb-loving Hispanics who dwell in the southern part of the state, some of whom apply decoctions of their beloved *Hediondilla* for ailments that might send others running for the Vicks VapoRub. They also use this tried old remedy to treat swollen feet, to ward off pneumonia, and to combat certain symptoms of "enfermedades Mexicanas" (diseases that official western medicine doesn't recognize), like one called "pasmo," which is said to result when an overheated body is chilled too suddenly.

There's no doubt about it: Southwesterners find much to endear the Creosote Bush to them, and not least of these is its reputed curative powers. The desert Indians, for whom the plant was also a good source of fuel, used a decoction of its olive-green leaves to purge their bodies of impurities, to heal their sores, to cure colds, to treat bowel complaints and delayed menstruation, and to ease indeterminate aches and pains of every variety. And although science doesn't substantiate any of their claims, some modern folk-healers still sing the praises of this historic old plant just as surely as the natives did, suggesting the use of Creosote tea for ailments that range from the common cold to cancer.

CURLY DOCK

Rumex crispus

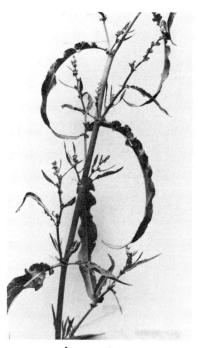

Curly Dock

Other names for Curly Dock: Other common names for this plant are Dock, Yellow Dock, Narrow Dock, and Sour Dock. To California's Hispanic population this herb is *Lengua de Vaca*. The Yuki Indians used to call it *O-pe-ol*.

Where to find it: You're as apt to find this native of Eurasia, Curly Dock, growing alongside some garbage-strewn street in the city slums as on some romantic overhang looking down upon the churning sea. It's especially fond of low places, clearings, sumps, ditches, meadows, and streamsides. It stays clear of altitudes over 9,000 feet, but otherwise it's never choosy; it's ever adaptable. Like the drab house sparrow, it's apt to be found most anywhere.

How to know it when you see it: This well-known old medicinal weed is easily identified by its big curly basal leaves, which are reminiscent of starched but unironed apron ruffles, and by its tall coffee-colored seedstalk, which is notably almost as familiar a sight in dry flower arrangments as it is on the shoulders of roads.

If they're of a good quality, the carrot-shaped roots, which are the dock's most medicinal part, are russet or brick-colored on the outsides, deep yellow or even orange within.

Its lore. Elsewhere on the continent, American Indians such as the Blackfeet and the Navajo used Curly Dock root decoctions to treat their own sores and the saddle sores of their horses, but like the Iroquois, the California tribes used it mostly as food. Toward the end of the nineteenth century, some of the Indians on the Round Valley Reservation in Mendocino County (probably the

Yukis, since it was they who'd given it an Indian name) were even cultivating the weed. This they did largely for its greens, but partly for its seeds from which, it's said, they made themselves a kind of mush.

It was the settlers who used Curly Dock as a medicine just as they had back east—or in their homelands across the sea—before ever they'd come to California. In those days *Rumex crispus* was a highly reputed medicine, not only to the doctoring housewife or the farmer in the barnyard, but even to genuine saddle-back doctors—those who'd actually been to school. The truth is that, until the 1890's, Curly Dock was firmly ensconced in the United States Pharmacopoeia. Even afterward it remained long respected.

It's true that if they'd had a choice in the matter—if there'd been enough doctors to go around—by the turn of the century many settlers would have chosen *not* to follow the old-fashioned advice of herbalists who bid them to depend on "Dr. Reason" and "Dr. Experience" rather than upon the trained physicians of the day. They had no choice, however, so they turned to those two inner healers and were led accordingly to tried old herbs like Curly Dock.

Used in the form of a boiled-root tea, this herb was believed beneficial as a spring tonic, a blood purifier, an appetite stimulator, a mild laxative, a digestive remedy, and as a treatment for rheumatism, lumbago, and jaundice. As a syrup, it was suggested for sore throats and coughs. In a leaf-poultice or a root salve, it was a medicine for human skin problems such as hives and ringworm and seven-year itches, not to mention mange on dogs and saddle sores on horses, donkeys, and mules.

Preparations derived from the potent root of the Curly Dock plant (infusions, syrups, and ointments much like those the oldtimers concocted) are used today by some modern-day herbalists and medicinal plant enthusiasts.

Warning: Since Curly Dock has been found to contain the principle oxalate, which can cause kidney damage if too much of the raw herb is consumed, it should not be used unless first well-cooked. In large quantities *raw* Dock and/or its uncooked derivitives may also cause nausea, vomiting, and diarrhea.

For some individuals, handling the leaves may cause skin irritation.

DEATH CAMAS

Zigadenus venenosus

Other names for the Death Camas: Another English name for this plant is Poison Camas. The Yuki Indian name for Death Camas was *Mas*. To many Pomos it was *Tsin*. The Wailakis called it *Ke-gus*.

Where to find it: This deadly poisonous member of the lily family is found on the coastline and in the mountains and forests in various locations. It favors rich meadows and the borders of creeks where it grows in the company of the true Camas, which is an edible plant and was once a staple food of the Indians.

How to know it when you see it: If you're a would-be wild food enthusiast as well as a votary of medicinal plants—beware. Don't even think of trusting yourself to know the difference between the bulb of the true Camas and that of the baneful *zigadenus*. This was a difficult feat even for the first Californians—they to whom rooting for bulbs was so much a way of life that the early settlers labeled them the "Digger Indians." These natives knew the features of the plants they sought as well as they knew the phases of the moon, and still, when it came to distinguishing the true Camas from Death Camas, once in a while they made a fatal mistake.

The trouble was that bulbs collected for consumption were dug up in late summer at a time when distinguishing earmarks were woefully few. Then the flowers were dead, the leaves were dried and sere, and all that was really left intact were those virtually identical onion-like bulbs, embedded side by side in the same moist habitat. It's much too easy for the collector, Indian, botanist, herbalist, or wild food enthusiast to mistake one for the other.

In springtime, when the plants are in bloom and the leaves are young, identification is not such a chore. The flowers of the true Camas, although occasionally whitish, generally tend toward shades of purple and blue. Those of its poisonous relative, great thick spikes of flowers, are best described as greenish-white. Sometimes reaching a height of three feet, the common Camas tends to be taller than its deadly kin, which ranges in size from one-half to two feet.

Its lore. The California Indians knew only too well that every single part of this plant was poisonous. They'd watched their kinsmen suffer from mistakenly sampling a bit of its bulb; they'd seen sheep expire just from munching its noxious leaves. They had every reason to detest the Death Camas, to shrink from it as they did from the cry of a screech owl, to shield their eyes at the sight of one spike of yellow-green flowers peering upward at the edge of some pond. But this too they knew: that which killed can also cure. And they took their cues accordingly. They cooked the bulbs of *Zigadenus venenosus,* and mashed them up to make poultices, which they applied externally to heal old sores, to ease the pain of rheumatism, and to relieve the discomforts of sprains and bruises. Poisonous though it was, it was good medicine, and in their wisdom they praised it unstintingly.

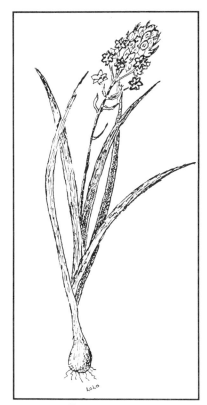

Death Camas

DIGGER PINE

Pinus sabiniana

Other names for the Digger Pine: This tree is also known as Nut Pine, Digger's Pine, and Digger Indian Pine. The Yuki Indian name for the tree was *Pol-cum ol*. To the Wailaki it was *Del shit*, whereas the Concow called it *Ta-ne*.

Where to find it: Most typical of the northern part of the state, in the old haunts of its namesake, the "Digger" Indian, this historic conifer is at home on dry slopes and ridges, in foothill woods, and on inner coastal ranges in many California locations.

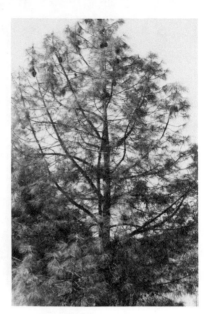

Digger Pine

How to know it when you see it: This homely native is sometimes a loner, sometimes a member of a small group of its ilk. Elsewhere it's found keeping company with the Manzanita or Common Blue Oak. Wherever it grows it's easily distinguished, even from a distance, by its sparse foliage and its wide-spreading, almost naked-looking branches.

The Digger Pine is by no means a typical conifer. It lacks the pole-like trunk, the forest-green color, the Christmas-tree shape, and the grace for which the typical pines are known. It's scraggly-looking, dull gray-green, with a sparsely-leafed crown that's sometimes as round and spreading as that of a broad-leaf genus. It's awkward as a teen-age boy, and short on shade.

The stiff needles of the Digger Pine, eight to ten inches long, are in bundles of three. The cones measure from five to eight inches long and have woody scales tipped with angular claws. The scaly bark ranges in color from black to terra cotta. The tree itself grows from forty to sixty feet tall and has a trunk (often forked) that ranges in size from one to two feet in diameter.

Its lore. The seeds of this homely conifer were such an important part of the diet of the so-called "Digger Indians" that the ever-labeling settlers named it, in turn, the "Digger Pine." In a sense it was fitting that they did, for this indeed was the "Digger's" tree—theirs for the taking, theirs for the using, but theirs too, most certainly, for their customary chants of thanks-giving for good food to eat.

Some thanks due the Digger Pine, however, were those it won for its medicinal uses, nearly as important to those namesake tribes as were the tasty little nuts they savored. It was its yellow pitch that they incorporated into their compendium of medicaments and used with full confidence. This substance sometimes served as a gum to chew for the relief of rheumatism; more often as a healing salve or a plaster for scratches, burns, sores, and splinters.

Seeing how effectively it worked for the Indians, some settlers made use of the Digger Pine's pitch as well, although they must surely have found its preparation tedious. To remove foreign substances, such as bits of bark, dirt, leaves or twigs, they'd probably employed much the same technique that's used by medicinal plant enthusiasts today. If so, they melted the gluey yellow substance at a low temperature and then poured it through a warmed colander or sieve, which was afterward nearly impossible to clean. They must have found it worth all the trouble, however, for after a time they devised even another usage for this healing exudation: a poultice made from a mixture of pitch and cornmeal, to be applied externally as a counterirritant for an assortment of internal maladies.

The settlers also visited the Digger Pine now and again for a store of its stiff gray-green needles from which to make a medicinal tea, an infusion reputed to prevent scurvy and/or serve as a mild diuretic. Insofar as it furnished leaves for this potion, the Digger Pine was no different than any other California pines or spruces or firs; they all had needles that served this purpose well. This was a fact which many miners, living in mortal fear of scurvy, were quick to take to heart. One such adventurer made a point of mentioning his first needle tea in a journal he penned about life in the California mines. "Had this evening spruce or fir tea for the first time," he wrote. "Some use it daily as a preventative of scurvy. It had to me a not very pleasant taste but think it is healthy. It makes a colorless tea, looks like water."

The Yokia Indians had yet another way of using the remarkably medicinal Digger Pine. They'd throw a pile of its twigs and leaves on the warm ashes of a dying fire, which had been built over rocks, and over which they'd sprinkle water from time to time. Then atop these ashes, a blanket-swathed patient, a victim of rheumatism, arthritis, or some other painful malady, would lie for several hours breathing the steam that rose up from the volatile oils.

Obviously, except for needle teas and bark infusions which were easy enough to make, Digger Pine remedies were both time consuming and messy. But this was all right with the early residents of California, for to their way of thinking, it was often the most painstaking treatment that best took away the pain.

DOG FENNEL

Anthemis cotula

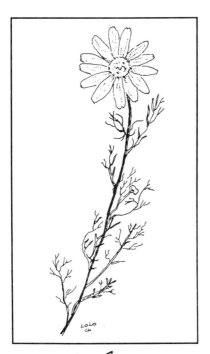

Dog Fennel

Other names for Dog Fennel: This invasive plant is also known as False Chamomile and Mayweed. The Yuki used to call it *Po-muk*.

Where to find it: This ill-smelling native of Europe is a common weed in all sorts of waste places from neglected front yards in city neighborhoods to open fields and vacant lots, throughout much of the state.

How to know it when you see it: If you see a plant from which even the chickens steer clear, which bees can't tolerate, and other plants shun, you've doubtless stumbled upon a dwelling place of the detestable Dog Fennel.

This plant is often mistaken for that most beloved of herbs, Roman Chamomile (*Anthemis nobilis*), which it does indeed resemble. It too is a member of the sunflower family. It too bears little daisy-like flowerheads with canary-yellow centers and petal-like ray flowers of purest white. It too, unjust as it may seem, is also called Chamomile. In fact, anyone unaware of its unpleasant odor and its weed-like traits might well describe Dog Fennel as "a pretty little flower."

Its lore. Native Californians knew from centuries of experience that bad tastes or bad odor in no way robbed a plant of its curative powers. As they saw it, even though they may have held their noses when they picked it, Dog Fennel was a very useful plant. Northern California Indians, suffering from colds and accompanying aches and pains, used to place the fresh plants in their bath water and then climb into this unlikely wash and soak their ailing bodies until the symptoms blessedly went away.

Though they may have spoiled the ambience of the kitchen in the process, even the early settlers made a cold medicine of the widespread Dog Fennel. By frying its reeky blossoms in a quantity of ordinary lard, they concocted an ointment that they used as an external application for sore throats and coughs.

How well these old weed remedies worked we cannot know. One thing, at least, is highly likely: colds probably didn't spread as fast when no one could tolerate getting close to the patient. It's said that even dogs can't stand Dog Fennel.

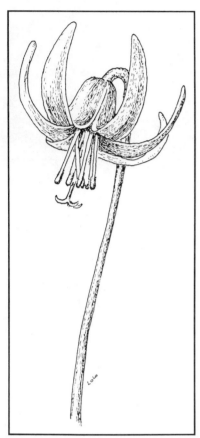

Dogtooth Violet

DOGTOOTH VIOLET

Erythronium grandiflorum

Other names for the Dogtooth Violet: Other English names for this plant are Fawn Lily, Trout Lily, Adder's Tongue, Leaf Adder, Yellow Fawn Lily, and Glacier Lily.

Where to find it: This legendary lily is found in open woods and moist meadows, in shady glens and in coniferous forests, by the sides of streams or near melting snowbanks at elevations up to 6,000 feet. Its favorite haunts are in the northern counties of Humboldt, Trinity, and Siskiyou.

How to know it when you see it: Look for a lily plant, from four to twelve inches tall, with two bright and shiny thick green leaves that sheath its naked stalks, and flowers whose sepals and petals are a matching golden-yellow. These early-spring bloomers are so markedly nodding, with their stalks bending like shepherds' crooks to bear them, it's as if they're peering down upon those shiny leaves, which in turn, appear to be pointing upward toward them.

Its lore. There's something about the Dogtooth Violet that gives rise to a sense of wonder in those who see it. Of course, it's probably because it blooms so early, because it shows its nodding face in March when all eyes are still eager to light on a flower—any flower at all—and no one can take a lily for granted even though it's less showy, less fragrant, less rare than its come-later kin. It makes sense. Spring spells newness and resurrection, and that's good cause for wonder.

But sometimes it seems that the Dogtooth Violet begets more awe than its share, as if it still possesses the powers for which the Wailaki Indians prized it so much, centuries ago. If it did—if it only did!—we could make of it a fine decoction, which could save us from danger in the woods where we walk. Don't the rattlesnakes abound there? Aren't they coiled up dreaming in our pathways even now? And isn't it true that their dreaming makes them nervous, and that in their agitation they may wake and strike at any moment? Can't we sense their movement as we hold our breaths and listen? Don't we know that death stalks us with every step we take, unless first we've washed our bodies in this marvelous decoction that stills the dreams of snakes and keeps them sleeping, sleeping soundly as we go walking by?

No other uses of the Dogtooth Violet were so dramatic as this one that stopped the dreams of snakes and kept the Wailakis safe. But this little lily did have other uses. The crushed corm made a fine poultice to heal boils, to smooth the skin, and to soothe the breasts of nursing mothers. And of course, then as now, its nodding yellow flowers were among the first to bloom in springtime, and that alone would have been just cause to hold this lily in esteem.

DOGWOOD

Cornus spp.

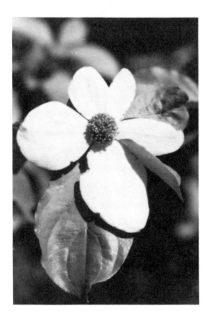

Dogwood

Other names for the Dogwood: Other English names for this lovely old medicinal are Flowering Cornel, Green Ozier, and Flowering Dogwood.

Where to find it: The familiar flowering dogwood is found growing all over the United States. Most California species seem to thrive best in shaded glens and by the sides of streams, although some are just as hale in tall forests where they fraternize with plants like Wax Myrtle, Salal, and Huckleberry, or in riverlands keeping company with Honeysuckle and Buttonbush and other such wildings.

How to know it when you see it: It's difficult to describe the Dogwood without calling on cliches, for this beautiful flowering hardwood is truly as American as Grandma's apple pie. As it happens, a description seems almost superfluous, for like the rose, and the apple pie too, for that matter, almost everyone knows it well already. For those who don't, however, some distinguishing details are in order.

The Dogwood is sometimes a shrub, sometimes a small tree that grows as tall as thirty feet. Its oval leaves, which appear as artistically arranged as if a florist's hand had put them in place, serve as a backdrop to its greenish-yellow flowers and lovely waxen-like, creamy-white bracts. Those leaves could be described as changelings, for as one season slips into another, they're transformed from typical deep green foliage to a purpled red, and at last, just before they drop from their branches, a rosy gold.

Its lore. The Dogwood, which is said to have the same soothing and healing properties as the ever-popular Chamomile, has figured, to some degree, in the folk medical practices of North Americans for many years. Sometimes, and in some places, it has been considered a medicament for the bowels. In other times and places it's counted as a substitute for Peruvian bark, of which Quinine is a notable derivitive. In California it's generally been regarded as a soothing, restorative tonic, good for the stomach, good for the spirit, almost as beneficial when simply gazed upon as when it's imbibed.

DOUGLAS IRIS

Iris douglasiana

Other names for the Douglas Iris: Other English names for this much-favored wildflower are Wild Iris, Fleur-De-Lis, and Flag. The Pomo Indians called this plant *Si-lim*. To the Yuki it was *Che-wish*, the Wailaki *Zhe-la-tsa-chit*.

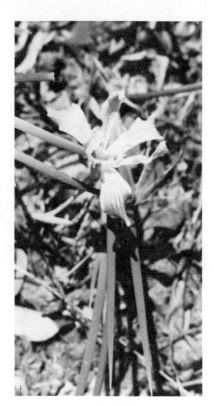

Douglas Iris

Where to find it: The Douglas Iris is found in a variety of California habitats: in coastal prairies, in mixed evergreen forests, on canyon floors, and in snow-melt gullies, but apparently its favorite spot is a grassy slope, where it thrives alongside grasses and sedges similarly inclined.

How to know it when you see it: This much-prized discovery of the nineteenth-century plant hunter, David Douglas, varies in color from pale cream to deep reddish-purple, with all shades of lavender in between. Sometimes reaching a height of three feet, it's often taller than similar species such as the Long-tubed Iris and Hartweg's Iris, which are rarely over two feet tall, or the Bowl-tubed Iris, which is even shorter. If you've come across the right specimen, then height can be a good clue to its identity and one perhaps more useful to the novice than one of its other earmarks: a floral tube and pedicel of approximately equal length.

Its lore. The Douglas Iris may have been used medicinally in much the same ways as its relative, the Rocky Mountain Iris, once considered a reputable treatment for such dissimilar ailments as jaundice and syphilis. But for the innovative young mothers of the Yokia Indian tribe, *Iris douglasiana* served another purpose entirely, and one so unique and valuable to them that it bears mention above all others. These women had to take their infants with them when they went trekking off into the hot, dry hillsides to pick the berries of the Manzanita. It could have been a miserable time for those little ones, for often the days were hot and the sun beat down relentlessly. Choking dust rose up like puffs of smoke and clung to faces wet with perspiration. Corners of eyes grew muddy, tempers short. Without proper protection, the babies might have suffered terribly. Instead they fared quite well, for their mothers had wrapped them up in the salvific green leaves of this lovely plant, a soft and pliant covering that retarded perspiration, saved them from thirst, and kept their plump little bodies cool.

DOUGLAS FIR

Pseudotsuga menziesii

Other names for the Douglas Fir: Other popular English names for this handsome tree are Douglas Spruce, Oregon Pine, and Fir. Yuki Indians called it *Nu*. To the Yokia it was both *Ka-la or na-ka* and *Na-ka*.

Where to find it: Another discovery of the nineteenth century naturalist, David Douglas (for whom the Douglas Iris was also named), this distinctive fast-growing tree is found in Yellow Pine and Redwood forests, in mixed evergreen woodlands, on moist slopes, and on coastal ranges at altitudes below 5,000 feet, in much of California.

How to know it when you see it: Look for a tree handsome enough to be considered an ornamental, with a shape and form just right for Christmas, and an air that declares it one of the most distinctive trees in the Pacific Northwest.

The needles of this important timber tree are about an inch and a half long, and stick out in all directions from its graceful, pendulous branches. When the tree is young its bark is grayish and smooth and marked with blisters of resin; older, it's furrowed and thick. The cones hang down and the twigs are pliant. The side branches of its conical crown are slightly weeping, lending it a ponderous look, an almost lordly bearing. In the moist coastal regions where it thrives the best, it's a big tree, measuring as much as eight feet in diameter, two hundred feet or more in height. Inland it's smaller, but wherever it grows it's lovely to see.

Its lore. Nowadays the Douglas Fir is best known for its beauty, its overall economic impact, and the role it plays in the reforestation projects that mean so much to the future of the land; all important features, not to be disdained. But once it was more; once it was medicine. Once the shaman gazed upon it with the focus of the healer, while some rheumatic tribesman or likewise-ailing woman eyed it with hope. In those days the Little Lake shamans deemed its needles better than Wormwood for a sweat-bath cure. Those pungent little leaves were tossed upon the fire, the proper prayers said, the right incantations mouthed, and in due course the pain itself, in some tangible form like that of a stone or a lizard or a frog, would be plucked forth from the ailing body so that health could be restored. The new spring buds of the Douglas Fir were also prized as medicine and used in a fine strong decoction intended to ease the woes of those dread venereal diseases that the white man had bequeathed to them.

The Shasta Indians had another interesting use for the Fir. At their funeral ceremonies they danced about the body of their deceased tribesfellow with staves of Fir clasped firmly in their hands and Fir branches attached to their bodies. Why Fir staves and Fir branches? What did this tree have to offer that others didn't? Was it the source of a kind of good luck charm? Or did it comprise a sort of preventive medicine? Or did it play both these roles simultaneously?

DUTCHMAN'S PIPE

Aristolochia californica

Other names for the Dutchman's Pipe: Other popular English names for this plant are Indian Root, Pipe Vine, and California Pipe Vine. Early Spaniards in California called it *Raiz del indio*.

Where to find it: This member of the Birthwort family, a relative of the better-known Wild Ginger, is found growing at altitudes below 1,500 feet on stream banks, in foothill woods and chaparral, on coastal ranges and in mixed evergreen forests in various California locations.

How to know it when you see it: Dutchman's Pipe is a perennial herb or shrub that twines or climbs, sometimes winding around or draping itself over other

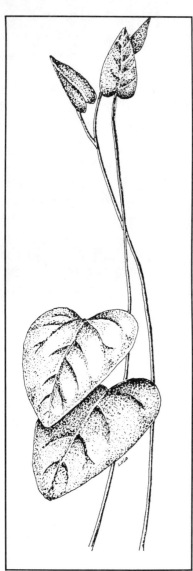

Dutchman's Pipe

shrubs with which it keeps company. It's a very easy genus to identify, so exotic looking, so outstandingly different, it catches the eye of the passerby and demands immediate attention. Hanging down from its winding branches, peering out from its typically-Birthwort, heart-shaped leaves, are its remarkable flowers. These blooms are so outlandishly devised it's as if they sprang forth from a dream, the dream of a pipe smoker perhaps, who fell asleep before the fireplace puffing on an old meerschaum pipe. That's what they most resemble, meerschaum pipes twisted, distorted, and dipped in pink paint.

Its lore. No herbals pay homage to this kin of Wild Ginger, nor does any field guide of medicinal wildings, nor treatise on useful plants of the west.

When it comes to acclaim as a medicinal plant, Dutchman's Pipe falls short nowadays, as if no one had ever prescribed it, applied it, or sang its praises. This is ironic indeed, for this remarkable vine is one of a genus that's long been perceived as medicinal. Consider, for example, its technical name, *Aristolochia*: clear testimony that once, elsewhere, it was regarded as a boon to women in the throes of childbirth. (*Aristos* is Greek for best; *locheia* means delivery.) California's Indians may not have used Dutchman's Pipe as a childbirth herb, but this old wilding figured prominently in their medical lore nonetheless.

According to Jose Longinos Martinez, who studied the flora and the fauna of Western Mexico, Old California (now called Baja California), and New California way back in 1792, the genus *Aristolochia* was the natives' much-prized "Indian Root," a widely-used and highly-respected remedy, which was dried, pulverized, and applied in the form of a powder to wounds and ulcers "in various states."

Apparently the most commonly used Indian Root was a species native to Mexico. Yet Martinez made a distinct point of mentioning that *Aristolochia* grew here too. He must have been referring to *A. californica*, better known as Dutchman's Pipe, which happens to be the only species found in California today. Why and how it fell from favor as a medicinal plant, we cannot know, but it seems more than fitting to reinstate it, to give it back its place in the history of the land.

ELDERBERRY

Sambucus spp.

Other names for the Elderberry: The various species of Elderberry are known as Blue Elderberry, Blue-Berry Elder, Red Elderberry, Red-Berry Elder, and Pacific Red Elder. Hispanic Californians call this plant *Sauco*. To the Cahuilla Indian it was *Hunqwat*.

Where to find it: The habitats of the various Elderberries differ considerably. *S. caerulea* is found in open places at altitudes up to 10,000 feet. *S. mexicana* is likely to be seen in Pinyon-Juniper woods in the mountains of the Mojave Desert. *S. callicarpa* favors damp woods and flats at low elevations. *S. microbotrys* is common in moist places at altitudes between 6,000 and 11,000 feet. Less common, *S. melanocarpa* is in habitats and at altitudes similar to those of *S. microbotrys*.

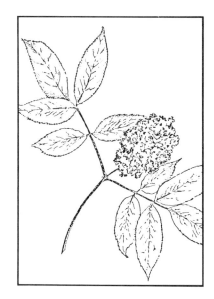

Elderberry

How to know it when you see it: *S. caerulea* is an erect shrub with a rather clumped appearance that grows to a height of twenty feet. Its saw-toothed leaves, each of which boasts from five to nine opposite-growing leaflets, are large and deciduous. Other California Elders, such as *S. callicarpa*, the Pacific Red Elder, which grows in damp woods and flatlands, attain tree size. *S. microbotrys* is a low shrub, as is *S. melanocarpa*.

Its lore. Most famous, perhaps, for the wine that's made from their delicious berries, or for their place in pies and other pastries, Elderberries have also played a substantial role in the folk medicine of California. To Indian and settler alike, the bark and root of the tree has been and still is considered diuretic, emetic, purgative; the leaves and shoots are diuretic; the flowers diaphoretic, the fruit aperient. Obviously then, one part or another of the plant has been used to treat a string of maladies that includes urinary problems, kidney complaints, edema, rheumatism, and constipation.

The desert tribes greatly prized the little Elderberry that shared their arid habitat, the white or blue-berried *S. mexicana* that grew blessedly near their village sites. This shrub has been described as a highly variable plant and one that's in need of study. Variable or not, it was apparently unwavering in its service as a source of basket dyes—bright yellows and oranges, deep purples and blacks—and a wellspring of priceless remedies. The desert Indians, for instance, brewed a fine tea from its blossoms and used it to treat stomach upsets, colds, fevers, flu, and other common complaints. This was a potion strong enough to serve the toughest chief, mild enough for a colicky baby mewling in his mother's arms, and good for the teeth of tribesfolk whatever their age or disposition.

The wood of the Elderberry was useful too. For the Yuroks, an Elder stick served as a kind of ruler with which to measure graves. To the Shastas it made a good knife for severing the naval cord of newborn infants. Why did Elder wood win out over that of other trees for the performance of these tasks? Was it simply a matter of convenience, a case of the ready accessibility of a particular genus? Or could it be that the Indians believed that this old medicinal plant possessed certain occult powers and/or medicinal properties that made it particularly fitting as an implement to prepare the Shastas for life on earth and the Yuroks for eternity?

Caution: Although the fruit of the Elderberry is nutritious, tasty, and safe to eat, especially when cooked, the roots, leaves, bark, and stems of the plant should never be consumed in any form, even as a tea. Cases of poisoning from this plant are rare, and yet the hazards are well worth noting. In fact, the hollow stems are so toxic that children who have fashioned them into whistles or blowguns are known to have suffered nausea and upset stomachs simply from having held them in their mouths.

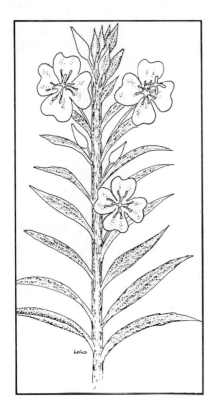

Evening Primrose

EVENING PRIMROSE

Oenothera clavaeformis, Oe. Hookeri, etc.

Other names for the Evening Primrose: The Spanish name for the Evening Primrose is *Flor de Santa Rita.* To the Cahuilla Indians it was *Tesavel.*

Where to find it: The Desert Primrose, from which the hungry Cahuilla used to collect both greens and caterpillars, prefers sandy plains and desert washes below 4,000 feet. Hooker's Evening Primrose, *Oe. Hookeri,* can be found in coastal scrublands and mixed evergreen forests, and other moist places in both southern and northern California at a variety of altitudes. In the marshy countryside around the little town of Forestville in Sonoma County, this plant grows as lush and thick as if someone was tending it with loving care.

How to know it when you see it: Most Evening Primroses have a stout, erect stem, alternate lancelike leaves, that grow smaller and smaller as they near its tops, and large four-petaled flowers that boom extravagantly all through the summer and fall. These showy blossoms appear almost luminescent by the light of the moon, when they're open wide for all the world to see. The stems of the well-known Hooker's Evening Primrose (*Oe. Hookeri*) are reddish, round, and slightly woolly, and the prominent mid-veins of its leaves are paler than the leaf itself, a kind of washed-out yellowish-lime color.

Its lore. Cahuilla Indians used the Desert Evening Primrose as a much-prized green and as the source of yet another viand they considered tasty: the caterpillar of the very moth that pollinates it, the *Celerio lineata,* which they named *Piy-akhtem.* But if they or any of the other Indian tribes ever used the plant medicinally, history is apparently silent on the subject. Nor do there seem to be any existing records to tell us what role it may have played in the early folk medicine of the first settlers in the state. Could it be that *Oenothera* belongs only to the herbal arts of the latter days? It's a certainty, at least, that here it shines. Today, even as wild-food enthusiasts serve its leaves as cooked greens and its roots as a stewing vegetable, modern California herbal buffs pay high prices for its precious oil, tout its use as an ingredient in a soothing cough syrup, as a mild laxative, as an anti-clotting agent, as a treatment for eczema, asthma, migraine headaches, and a long list of allergic conditions.

FENNEL

Foeniculum vulgare

Other names for Fennel: Other popular English names for Fennel are Sweet Fennel and Wild Anise. The Spanish name for the plant is *Hinojo.*

Where to find it: An old-world plant belonging to the carrot family, Fennel has become extensively naturalized in various locations throughout the state. At first, more abundant in the southern and central sections, it's now a familiar plant in much of northern California as well. In fact, its lacy yellow umbels are such a common sight along the freeways and backroads of North Bay counties nowadays it's hard to believe they weren't there before the roads were, that they didn't wave in the winds in the days when a widow woman named Maria arrived there footweary, with her clan of fatherless children, and built the Carrillo adobe: the first house ever to dot the Santa Rosa plain.

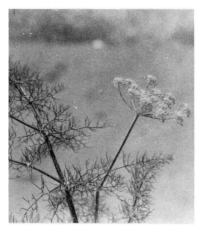

Fennel

How to know it when you see it: It's not hard to identify this graceful perennial herb. You may recognize it even before you see it if you catch a waft of its sweet, enticing odor, reminiscent of candy counters where a penny bought a licorice stick, a nickel bought a whole bag full. As to its appearance, its stems are cane-like and tall; its leaves as lacy as a Spanish *chalina* (scarf). When it first blooms in springtime, its display—compound umbels of tiny flowers—is modest enough, but as time passes on and summer settles in, more and more of these flat-topped clusters appear atop the waxen stems like so many yellow doilies put there to dress up the countryside. By mid-August they're so abundant it's as if some mad tatter can't stop her shuttle, can't tie off her thread, and won't quit tatting 'til California's covered with her tracery.

Its lore. Like other Americans of the day, those who roved westward in the 1800s looked upon themselves as a new breed of humanity, people caught up in the spirit of growth and development that seemed almost to crackle in the air around them. Times were changing. Steamboats were sailing the rivers back home in the east; miners there were using safety lamps; pianists were keeping time with metronomes; some people back in civilized territory even owned a clever little gadget called a kaleidoscope. California, of course, was devoid of these wonders, a wilderness yet to be tamed. But the people who'd come to tame it thought of themselves as knowing and wise, free of the past and all its silly shackles. It's true that they still made their own herbal remedies to treat their ills. They had no choice; store-bought decoctions were not to be had. They'd known this beforehand, of course. They'd come westward with seed. But as they cultivated backyard herbs, foraged for wild ones, and dried, measured, pulverized, and decocted them, they cast aside some of the superstitions that had surrounded them. Gone were the days, for example, when it was believed that Fennel improved the eyesight of snakes and that, therefore, on those grounds alone, it was good for the human eye as well. Ironically, however, they continued to use the herb for their eyes. The only difference was that now they did so with no grounds at all.

Whether snakes like Fennel or not, and whether or not it's foolish to think that they do or they don't, it's interesting to note that some modern Californians, like herb enthusiasts elsewhere, still use Fennel-seed tea as an eyewash. A similar infusion is used to relieve stomach-aches and cramps, to soothe infant colic, to ease flatulence, and to promote lactation in nursing mothers.

Like the survivalists and wild-food enthusiasts who make soups and salads from its leaves and stems and roots, even the most conservative of modern herbalists tout this graceful plant for its proven antispasmodic properties, its high content of calcium, potassium, iron, vitamins A and C, and its traces of protein and phosphorus.

FIGWORT

Scrophularia californica

Other names for the Figwort: Other popular English names for Figwort are California Figwort, Scrofula Plant, and Carpenter's Square. The Wailaki Indians called this plant *Wa-cha*.

Where to find it: Found from the Santa Monica Mountains north to British Columbia, California Figwort is a common plant in damp places, especially in thickets.

How to know it when you see it: This relative of the highly poisonous Foxglove is an extremely variable plant, often not easy to identify. Generally it's rather weedy looking, has coarse stems, bears leaves that are triangular and serrated, and ranges from three to six feet in height. Its short tubular flowers, reddish-brown in color, bear two projecting upper petals.

Its lore. There was a time when California Figwort was a vital source of salt to the Yuki and the Wailaki Indians of Northern California. These tribes were herbivorous; they had to have this mineral in their diet in order to maintain their health. Yet it wasn't easy for them to obtain it. They couldn't travel freely to the salt-rich coast, as other tribes could, for they were hemmed in by a veritable wall of enemies. This is not to say that they lacked the verve to fight for the necessities of life. In the old days, many a salt supply (such as one that was located at Stony Creek in Colusa County) was the scene of skirmishes and confrontations between one desperate people and another. But there was a safer way to acquire this vital commodity; the natives could turn to plants like Figwort, which was itself a good source. It was not an instant supplier, however. They had first to roll the fresh green leaves of the plant into little balls, dry them thoroughly, set them atop a rock, and bake them in a small fire until they were reduced to salty ashes.

The settlers had other ways of using this plant, especially those who still clung to the concept of the Doctrine of Signature, that old belief that each plant bears some sign that tells the world of its intended usage. The leaves and the roots of Figwort are covered with nodes, and, to these believers, this was certain testimony that here was an herb meant to treat eruptions of the skin.

Figwort is still in use today. Even herbalists who don't abide by the Doctrine of Signatures, who see it as both superstitious and reactionary, suggest the use of this herb as a remedy for the same skin disorders that it used to treat, ailments that ranged from athlete's foot to diaper rash.

FREMONT COTTONWOOD

Populus fremontii

Other names for the Fremont Cottonwood: Other common English names for this tree are Aspen and Cottonwood. The Yuki Indians called it *Pat-mil*. To the Cahuilla it was *Lavalvanat*.

Where to find it: This handsome Californian, which is more common to the southern part of the state than to the northern, thrives in moist places below 6,500 feet. On canyon floors—one of its favorite habitats—it's often found in the company of Oregon Ash, Big Leaf Maples, and Live Oaks. In another of its haunts, streamside, it's apt to be seen with Water Birches, or its kin, the fragrant Black Cottonwood.

How to know it when you see it: The leaves of Fremont Cottonwood, which lie somewhere between heart-shaped and triangular, are shiny and green, coarsely toothed, and yellow-stemmed. The deeply-furrowed bark of old trees is brick red or deep russet, while that of younger specimens is smooth, thin, and grayish brown. A rapidly-growing, broad-crowned shade tree, it ranges in height from 50 to 75 feet and measures 2 to 5 feet in diameter.

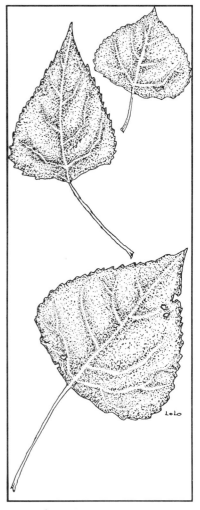

Fremont Cottonwood

Its lore. The role played by the Fremont Cottonwood in the folk medicine practices of early Californians seems unimpressive when compared to that of many other medicinal plants growing wild across the land. It was never a popular remedy with settlers. Early explorers and naturalists who described it rarely honed in on its use as a remedy. It was never touted widely in nineteenth-century herbals. Most modern field guides of medicinal plants fail to give it mention at all. The trouble is that the people who *did* consider it medicinal and used it accordingly, and may conceivably have done so effectively for many centuries, were not the ones who wrote herbals or kept journals or sent data about the California flora to dignitaries elsewhere. They were Indians, the first Californians, and to them the Fremont Cottonwood was well worth using as a remedy. They employed its leaves to make a poultice to ease away muscle strain.

From leaves and bark both they concocted a lotion with which they soothed their headaches. They made a bark decoction, which they employed not only to soothe and heal their own cuts and bruises but to treat the sores of their horses. And in those days, when veterinary practice was every man and woman's business, a medicinal plant that was effective for both humans and equines was highly prized indeed.

FRENCH MARIGOLD

Tagetes patula

Other names for the French Marigold: Another English name for *Tagetes patula* is Deer Herb. The early Spanish Californios called this plant *Hierba del venado*.

Where to find it: *Tagetes patula* is a native of Mexico that has become naturalized in Santa Barbara, where it resides in vacant lots and dumps.

How to know it when you see it: This sunny alien bears branching stems that are often purple-tinted, sharply-toothed leaves, showy disk flowers, and rays of matching yellowish-orange.

Its lore. There are so many uncertainties, so many unsolved mysteries, surrounding the long-forgotten deer herb that its inclusion in this compendium has to rest, in part, on circumstantial evidence. This is ironic indeed, for if the evidence is sound, there was a time when it was one of the most popular medicinal herbs abounding in that wilderness called "the Californias." In fact, after his 1792 expedition into that bear-infested territory, the venturesome "natural philosopher," Jose Loginos Martinez, placed *haierba del venado*, a "strong stomach stimulant," near the top of a list of "the medicinal herbs most frequently found and used" there.

One problem lies in the fact that although this plant does grow wild in California now, albeit in a very limited area, it was not growing north of the border when Martinez made his observations. (In point of fact, there was no border then; that was twelve years before the official demarcation of Alta and Baja California.) The herb was one that we would now term "a native plant of Mexico." Therefore, along the same line of thinking, the natives who used it were "the Indian tribes of Mexico," whose folk medicine theoretically became separate from ours as soon as borders were established. This doesn't mean, however, that the deer herb failed to figure in the folk medicine of this more northerly land as well. As it happened, its acceptance here was ultimately dependent, not upon the Indians who first used it, but upon the Spanish settlers who made New California their home, many of whom enthusiastically endorsed the popular Indian herbs of *both* the Californias.

It's a certainty that barter and trade of medicinal herbs—dried plants, seeds, seedlings and cuttings—was a common practice with Spaniards all up and down that borderless land. It's equally certain that some Spanish settlers in New California, most especially the mission padres, husbanded extensive gardens in which they grew many of the native plants of Mexico. Records show that some of the Indians' favorite medicinals, like Canchalagua and Indian Fig, were much-prized by the Spanish settlers of both Californias, especially by the mission priests who so often had to double as doctors to their enormous flocks. Did they also treasure *Tagetes*? It seems highly probable that they did. And since *Tagetes patula*, a native of Mexico, now grows wild within the state, although, notably, only in Santa Barbara, it would be folly to exclude it simply because descriptions of old California gardens fail to mention it specifically.

It's interesting to note that the single habitat in which this old medicinal plant grows wild within the state was once the home of one of the mission padres who would have been most apt to cultivate it in his gardens. This was the remarkable Father Luis Gil Y Taboada, a priest at Santa Barbara Mission in the early 1800s who, more than any other of his ilk, made a sizable contribution to the medical lore of California. Born in Mexico, so deeply involved with the Indians he served that he learned to speak their tongue, he was always interested in the healing arts. A self-styled physician, he not only performed the first Caesarian operation in California (an enormous feat in a frontier land, in a day and age when the procedure was far from commonplace anywhere in the world), but later became head of California's first hospital, the so-called *asistencia* of San Rafael. It takes only a small leap of the imagination to fancy that the good padre cultivated the deer herb while he was in Santa Barbara, that it escaped from the mission gardens to flourish unnoticed in the vicinity for many years until at last one day, decades later, someone wondered at a marigold blooming incongruously among the rubble at the dump.

It's a fascinating conjecture—but nothing more. Father Gil Y Taboada may or may not have prescribed this little marigold for the ailing flock who came to him for help. One way or the other, there's no scientific basis whatever for connecting this unsung man of yesterday's Santa Barbara to the long-forgotten Mexican herb that grows wild in that same city today. There are, however, good grounds to pluck these two out of the no-man's-land of forgotten plants and forgotten people and give back to each of them a justified place in the rich folk history of California.

GIANT BLAZING STAR

Metzelia laevicanlis

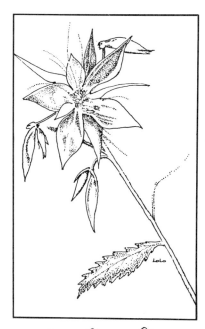

Giant Blazing Star

Other names for the Giant Blazing Star: Another popular English name for this plant is Star Flower. The Wailaki called it *Ka-tsak-u*. Its Little Lake name was *Ek*.

Where to find it: Growing at altitudes below 8,500 feet, the Giant Blazing Star is much at home in old dried stream beds and in disturbed places where the earth is rocky and stony. In some parts of the state such as Trinity County, where it's as familiar a sight as wild fuchsia and Pennyroyal, it's frequently seen blooming right beside the highways, a pleasure to travellers passing through in the morning before its showy blooms have closed up shop for the day.

How to know it when you see it: "Giant," of course, is the key word to the identification of this great showy biennial, a late summer bloomer and a member of the *Loasa* family. A coarse plant and a stout one, its hollow stem, white as sun-blanched bone, sometimes reaches a height of five feet. Its night-blooming star-like flowers of pale yellow measure from four to six inches wide. Its big elongated, triangular leaves, which stick as tenaciously as strips of velcro to the clothing of passersby, are grayish in color and raggedly toothed.

Its lore. Although it's not a particularly impressive sight at high noon, when evening comes along the Giant Blazing Star is one of those flowers that's bound to capture the eye and the imagination. In the old days, before television came and changed the world, when dusk was still a time for outdoor games, the Indian children used to gather around it and wait breathlessly for the moment that its pale yellow petals would begin to unfold. They called it simply the "star flower," and surely that's how they perceived it when they let their fancies flow: as a star that had dropped directly out of the heavens just to shine on them.

The adults too admired the Giant Blazing Star, and not only for the show it put on when the sun went down, but for the role it played in keeping them well. From its great "sticky" leaves, they made a fine decoction, which was a remedy for stomach-aches when taken internally, a medicine for skin diseases when applied externally as a wash. Notably, this medicament was still in use as late as a hundred years ago.

GOLDENROD

Solidago californica

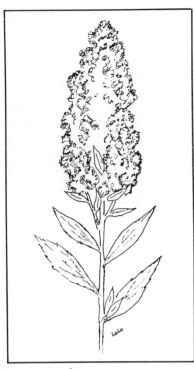

Goldenrod

Another name for the Goldenrod: The Cahuilla name for the California Goldenrod was *Pa'kily.*

Where to find it: Adaptable to either moist or dry places, the California Goldenrod, *Solidago californica,* is common in fields, clearings, and woodland glens, at altitudes ranging from 200 to 7,500 feet in many and varied locations throughout the state.

How to know it when you see it: The California Goldenrod bears a thick, short, and spiky cluster of showy yellow flowerheads which often grow in clumps. Its leaves, dark green in dry mountain locations, are greyish when it's found near the coast. The plant ranges in size from one to four feet.

Its lore. Records of the medicinal use of Goldenrod by the original Californians are surprisingly sketchy, especially in light of the fact that one species or another of *Solidago* had wide Indian usage in other parts of North America. It is known, however, that the Cahuilla Indians turned to this herb for the ingredients of both a hair rinse and a medicament for feminine hygiene.

As to the early settlers, since there was a time when even American physicians approved the use of Goldenrod leaves as a diuretic and a carminative, these newcomers must certainly have included *S. californica* in their compendium of household cures.

GOOSEBERRY

Ribes californicum

Other names for the Gooseberry: The Yuki Indian name for the California Gooseberry was *Gol-le.* The Pomo called it *Lom,* whereas the Yokia name was *Ta-ra-tit.*

Where to find it: Happy in locations less than 2,500 feet above sea level, the California Gooseberry thrives in many habitats. It's found in rocky canyons, alongside roadways, on open slopes, in Redwood forests, in foothill woods, on coast ranges, and in mixed evergreen forests from Mendocino County to Monterey.

How to know it when you see it: This attractive shrub, as beautiful as the lovliest of fuchsias, according to the naturalist, Douglas, who wrote about it in

1832, is intricately branched, and bears flowers that range from greenish-white to purplish, and light-red bristled fruit.

Its lore. It's probable that berries have never been more important to any group of people on earth than they once were to the California Indians. Eating them, which was always a delight and a pleasure, was sometimes a necessity. Picking them was an occupation, a cause for celebration, almost a way of life; and yet these original Californians rarely looked upon the Gooseberry as a remedy. That viewpoint was to be assumed by the herb-dependent American settlers, individuals who'd been schooled either by the Indians elsewhere (some of whom did indeed consider the Gooseberry medicinal) or by herbalists of the day, whose opinions they'd read or heard and taken to heart. As they perceived it, Gooseberries promoted a flow of urine, helped fevers drop, improved the appetite, soothed attacks of malaria, eased seizures, quenched the thirst, broke up kidney stones, gave comfort to pregnant women, and helped cure canker sores.

GOOSE GRASS

Polygonum aviculare

Other names for Goose Grass: Other popular English names were Knotweed, Knotgrass, Common Knotweed, Ninety-Knot, Centinode, Allseed, Swynel Grass, Redrobin, Pig Rush, Bird's Tongue, and Beggarweed.

Where to find it: Originally from Eurasia, this familiar annual can be found growing all over California. Look for it on beaches and salt marshes near the coast, in alkaline soil in interior locations, and in dooryards and vacant lots in cities and towns across the state.

How to know it when you see it: First of all, Goose Grass is not really a grass at all. Nor is it a small legume, as it's sometimes thought to be. Its technical name, *Polygonum*, which is Greek for "many knees," affords a good clue to its prime identifying feature, the many joints with stipules surrounding the stem above the joints. Look for all those "knees" on a plant that's thriving in heavily trafficked places where the ground is hard-packed and grass can't survive. Then look for simple leaves (instead of the leaflets of the legume it's sometimes thought to resemble) on short, slender, bluish-green stems, and tiny red or rose-margined flowers, and you've doubtless stumbled across that hearty member of the Buckwheat family best known in California as Goose Grass, a favorite viand not only of geese but of cows, chickens, and countless wild birds.

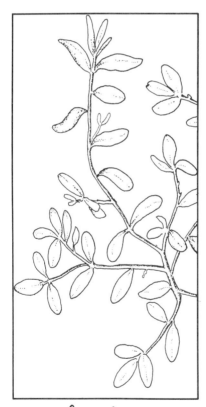

Goose Grass

Its lore. This weed, which Shakespeare called "the hindering knotgrass," was once believed to stunt the growth of both the farm animals and the youngsters whose very tromping feet had hard-packed the soil and rendered it just right for the plant to burgeon forth. That was a reputation it didn't deserve, however, for insofar as the workings of the human body are concerned, Goose Grass appears to be a most beneficent herb. Squirt its juice in the nostrils of a nosebleeder, it's said, and the bleeding stops at once. And a tea of the plant is a worthy old folk remedy: good for diarrhea, bleeding piles, and hemorrhages of every sort.

In the late 1800s the Mendocino County Indians and neighboring settlers used to make a concoction of the whole Goose Grass plant plus a quantity of oak bark, and use this mixture as an effective astringent. Even more importantly, a similar potion was sometimes administered as a substitute for quinine. In that time and place, the ubiquitous Goose Grass was better known as a healing medicament than as the "hindering knotgrass" that the bard had perceived it to be, or the ugly weed it's often considered today.

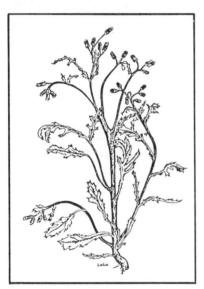

Groundsel

GROUNDSEL

Senecio vulgaris

Another name for Groundsel: Life Root.

Where to find it: Introduced from Europe, strictly by accident, this common weed, a member of the composite family, has become naturalized all over Canada and the United States. Fast-growing and rapidly-spreading, it is found firmly ensconced in gardens, fields, vacant lots, and almost anywhere else where the earth has been disturbed.

How to know it when you see it: A homely little annual, a popular food for canaries, a pesky weed to gardeners, Groundsel is a low-growing plant with greenish-purple stems ranging in height from six to twelve inches. Its greyish-green leaves are narrow, oblong, and so jaggedly lobed as to appear unkempt and ragged. Its flowerheads, too, are somewhat less than beauteous; tubular-shaped, yellow, and completely rayless, they give the impression of being not quite finished.

Its lore. Groundsel earns mention on these pages not so much for the role it's played in California lore but for its place in folk medicine in general all over the world. An herb that's been considered a valuable remedy for hundreds, possibly even thousands, of years, and that happens to flourish all over the state, just can't be ignored.

In the past, Groundsel concoctions of one variety or another (including an herb and wine beverage and a popular poultice made of bruised fresh Groundsel and breadcrumbs) have been used to treat an assortment of ailments, among them stomach-aches, nervousness, intestinal problems, toothaches, disturbances of the pelvic organs, boils, chapped hands, and sore eyes. Nowadays the herb has fallen into comparitive disuse, its purported virtues minimized, its supposed cures debunked and discounted. But once it was a much-prized cure-all. Once, even the Roman naturalist, Pliny, sang its praises.

And notably, there are still a few herbalists in California and elsewhere who echo his song today.

GREEN AMARANTH

Amaranthus spp.

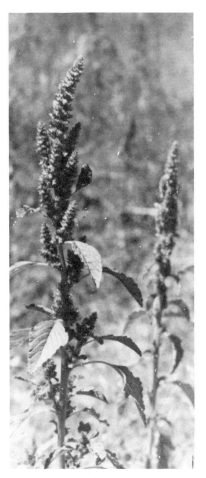

Green Amaranth

Other names for the Green Amaranth: Other popular English names for this plant were Red Cockscomb, Coxcomb, Love-Lies-Bleeding, Pigweed, Alegria, Velvet Flower, and Prince's Feather. The Cahuilla Indian name for one species of *Amaranthus*, *A. fimbriatus*, was *Pekat*.

Where to find it: A lover of vacant lots, Green Amaranth often grows so thickly there it's as if it aims to crowd out the "for sale" signs that have a way of sprouting up in the very same habitats. This old medicinal herb is found in waste places all over the state, just as it's found in similar spots in other states and other countries.

How to know it when you see it: Perhaps most typical of the *Amaranthus* species growing in California is *Amaranthus retroflexus*, best known as Green Amaranth, a native of tropical America which grows, with surprising rapidity, to a height of five feet. If you suddenly notice an enormous population of sprightly-looking, lettuce-green weeds growing profusely in a vacant lot where you'd swear there was no such thing a week ago, chances are your eyes have lit upon a new upcropping of the hearty Green Amaranth, one species of a plant that's been used medicinally for hundreds of years.

The most outstanding feature of the Green Amaranth is its many spikes of chaffy little flowers. These blooms are as vibrant a green as its leaves when the plant is young, but reddish in maturity, as are its older stems. Red too is its rather lovely root, which looks like a sculpting of a garden carrot executed incongruously in the finest porcelain and dipped in a rose-colored wash.

The leaves of this plant, suede-like to the touch, are greyish-green on the underside, almost chartreuse on top. The stems, practically purplish at the base, are round, slightly ridged, and filled with a pith as green as only a Green Amaranth can be.

Its lore. Today Amaranth is a plant which might best be described as "a mild astringent," used most often in leaf-tea form, or in a decoction made of one ounce of herb to one pint of boiling water. It's considered a good herb for the mucous membranes, a worthy treatment for slight stomach irritations, a remedy for diarrhea, and a nice innocuous tonic for recuperating flu victims. But back in the days when the famous herbalist, Nicholas Culpeper, was busy mixing his potions in the London apothecary, where he plied his trade, the properties of this herb were perceived as considerably more powerful. One species was even a "gallant anti-venereal," and a remedy for the dread French pox.

To the early settlers in California this herb was still looked upon as a most beneficent medicinal plant, perhaps not so powerful as Culpeper figured, but certainly a boon in the doctorless wilderness of the far, far west.

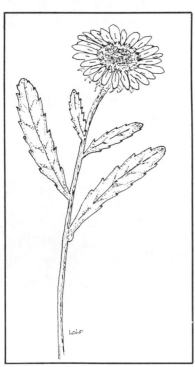

Gumplant

GUMPLANT

Grindelia spp.

Other names for Gumplant: Other popular English names for this plant were Grindelia, Gum Plant, Gumweed, Rosinweed, Resin Weed, and Tarweed. The Pomo Indians called it *She-na-tik*. To California's hispanics it is *Yerba del Buey*.

Where to find it: There are several species of Gumplant growing in California. Probably the most commonly known of these are the Great Valley Gumplant, Puget Sound Gumplant, Coastal Gumplant, and the Idaho Resin Weed. Great Valley Gumplant (*Grindelia camporum*) loves dry fields and open spots like vacant lots and rocky roadsides. Puget Sound Gumplant (*G. integrifolia*) is found near the coast, from San Francisco north to British Columbia. Coastal Gumplant (*G. latifolia*) likes habitats similar to those of the Puget Sound species, but its range is from San Francisco south to Santa Barbara. Like the Great Valley Gumplant, the Idaho Resin Weed (*G. nana*) dwells in dry fields and other open places.

A common westerner, *Grindelia* is notably one of the very first plants to sprout up in disturbed places such as vacant lots and roadsides, dooryards, and fields. It's also found in salt marshes and on foothills and slopes.

How to know it when you see it: Aster-like members of the sunflower family, Gumplants are coarse and resinous perennials, bearing large, sunny yellow flowerheads, and ray flowers at the tips of their branches. The alternate leaves, pale green, leather-like, and somewhat rigid, are usually serrated and sessile, often clasping as well. The Great Valley Gumplant reaches four feet in height, whereas the other species named above rarely exceed three. All species exude a sticky and balsamic "milk," for which they're appropriately named Gumplant. All are fairly conspicuous, easy to spot, generally easy to identify.

At close range the Gumplant is not a pretty flower, not the sort of plant to be cultivated in the garden for anything other than medicinal purposes. From a distance, however, it can be a cheering sight, especially in August, when it's still blooming lustily after so many other flowers have wilted and fallen into the dust.

Its lore. Although it wasn't introduced into the commercial drug trade until late in the 1800s, long after the California settlers had discovered its virtues, Gumplant is considered by many herbalists to be the single most important medicinal plant in the state. Its fame, which began with the Indians who used it as a blood purifier and a cure for colds and colic, has far exceeded the bounds of the state, however. It's an official drug plant in European medicine. It's lauded by herbalists all over the world, featured in many an herbal and field guide, and widely used as a remedy for an ongoing list of physical complaints including bladder infections, bronchitis, asthma, nervousness, and stomach disorders. The crushed flowers, which the Indian children once chewed like gum, are sometimes used as a poultice for the treatment of Poison Oak, minor burns, and slow-healing sores. And Gumplant leaf or flower tea, which some find as tasty as any teas on the market, is reputedly excellent for hacking coughs.

HONEYSUCKLE

Lonicera spp.

Other names for Honeysuckle: Other popular English names were Honeysuckle Vine and Honey Vine. The Yuki Indian name for this plant was *Hi-wat*.

Where to find it: Honeysuckle is most at home on dry slopes at altitudes from 1,000 to 6,000 feet. Look for it too in chaparral, alongside streams, in foothill woods, on brushy slopes, and in Yellow Pine forests. You'll find it blooming from May to July.

How to know it when you see it: The Honeysuckle is a familiar twining shrub, sometimes erect, sometimes sprawling, climbing this way and that way over the other plants with which it keeps company. It has slender stems, opposite leaves, and fragrant yellow flowers.

Its lore. From those halcyon times when the Indian children were the only youngsters in the land, 'til now when the towns are teeming, this native shrub has long been beloved by the boys and girls of California. So it is with children everywhere that the plant is known. It's fun to suck the nectar from the long yellow Honeysuckle flowers. Adult Indians found other uses for this lovely plant. Its long flexible stems were useful to basket weavers; its leaves made an excellent lotion with which to soothe sore eyes.

Today some herbalists use the Honeysuckle flowers to concoct a syrup for bronchitis and asthma, and the bark to make a lotion for the skin, a gargle for sore throats, and a cream for the complexion.

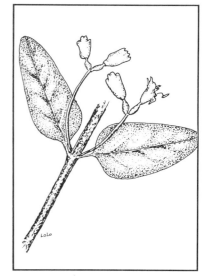

Honeysuckle

HOP

Humulus lupulus

Other names for Hop: Other popular English names for this plant were Hops and Common Hop.

Where to find it: Originally cultivated for brewing purposes (as in Sonoma County where it was once of considerable economic importance), the Hop vine escaped from the fields where it was cultivated and is now naturalized in several California locations.

How to know it when you see it: This native plant of Eurasia is a perennial vine that sometimes grows to lengths of thirty feet. Its stems are rough; its opposite leaves are three-lobed; its fruiting cones (strobiles), which contain the valuable bitters for which the plant is prized, are covered with yellowish glands.

Its lore. The Hop vine had already escaped from cultivation by the 1890s, and was, in fact, by then a respected remedy of the Indians and settlers who dwelt in Mendocino County. It was the prime ingredient (sometimes the only ingredient) of a comforting poultice, which was applied to sprains, bruises, and swollen ankles.

Modern herbalists have other uses for this twining vine with the odd-shaped strobiles. A strong Hop tea is said to ease restlessness, relieve insomnia, lessen the effects of delirium tremens, reduce fever, and soothe a vast assortment of vexing aches and pains. It is an herb that years haven't robbed of glory at all; it's still well-respected, a boon to insomniacs from every walk of life. Even some of the most pragmatic pharmacologists afoot are apt to praise it for its sedative effects.

HOREHOUND

Marrubium vulgare

Other names for Horehound: Other popular English names for this plant were Soldier Tea, Common Horehound, Marrubium, Marvel, White Horehound, and Horehound Mint. The Spanish name for Horehound plant is *Marrubio*.

Where to find it: A native of Europe, the Horehound escaped from cultivation many years ago and is now naturalized in various locations throughout the west. Preferring open ground and dry waste places, it thrives, weed-like, along roadsides and in old neglected fields.

How to know it when you see it: Fuzzier than the upper lip of a teenage boy, the erect stems of the Horehound plant, branching out from the plant's base, bear opposite, hairy-topped leaves that are much-crinkled and scalloped, and oval or roundish in shape. The flowers are usually white or the palest of light lavenders and grow in pincushion-like circles around the square stem, just above the point at which the opposite leaves appear to meet.

Its lore. Although the Horehound plant had already escaped from cultivation by the 1900s, and was so well-established by then as to be considered a common weed in some parts of the state, it was never a favorite medicinal plant of the California Indians. Some of them tried it, of course; there were always a few who were eager to experiment with the newcomers' remedies, just as there were always newcomers ready to sample theirs. But generally speaking, the Horehound was looked upon as a settler's herb, as beloved and necessary to them as it had been to their grandparents.

It was not surprising that Americans and Europeans brought Horehound with them when they came to California. In their day, as all through the nineteenth century, the plant was still looked upon as the cure-all it had been considered when the great Roman naturalist, Pliny, was penning its praises. There was scarcely an herbalist of the 1800s who didn't tout it as highly as he had.

At one time or another during its long and colorful history, Horehound has been used as treatment for a list of physical complaints, including snakebite (for which Pliny considered it an excellent antidote), constipation, "female problems," diarrhea, nervousness, insomnia, sore throat, jaundice, dyspepsia, hysteria, poor appetite, colds, and chest congestion. The California settlers used it primarily as a treatment for colds and diarrhea (for which they decocted a variety of syrups and strong leaf teas) or as an ingredient in the once popular Horehound-candy cough drops, so dear to the children of the nineteenth and early twentieth centuries.

HORSETAIL

Equisetaceae equisetum

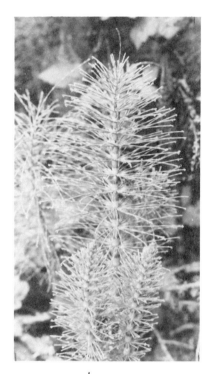

Horsetail

Other names for Horsetail: Other popular English names for this plant were Field Horsetail, Scouring Rush, Dutch Rush, Devil's Guts, Pewterwort, Bottlebrush, Shave brush, Shave Grass, Joint-Grass, Joint Weed, Pipes, and Bull Pipes. The Yuki Indian name for the Horsetail was *Shan-tum*. The Little Lake called it *Shu-me*.

Where to find it: This fascinating spore-producing plant is found on roadsides, by shaded brooks, near mountain streams, and in swampy spots in many Northern California locations.

How to know it when you see it: Like a character in a fairy tale, a prince, perhaps, who's haplessly transformed into a frog, the Horsetail plant appears entirely different at one time than it does at another. Unless forewarned, a novice in the field is apt to be deceived. In early springtime the hollow stems of the plant, which rise up from the moist soil like tiny bamboos, are multi-jointed, and completely unbranched. The top of each of these ends in a kind of cone where the reproductive cells (the spores) of the plant are produced. Later on in the season these fruiting stems all wither away, only to be replaced by new ones that are as profusely branched as they were formerly naked, thick with whorls of green. It's then that a stand of Horsetail plants takes on the appearance of a miniature pine forest, a delight to the eyes of imaginative children, or adults who still know how to let their fancies fly.

Crystals of silica are formed on these plants, rending them excellent contrivances for scouring pots and pans. Hence, they're called scouring rushes almost as often as they're called Horsetails. One way or the other, they're as much a part of Northern California as the Redwood forests or the pounding surf.

Its lore. Probably the most unusual medicinal use to which the Horsetail was ever put in California was at the hands of the Indian shaman as a means of revitalizing patients to whom normal vigor was somehow lost. Properly primed with prayer and fasting, visions and dreams, the medicine doctor—oftentimes a woman—would toss the hollow stems of *Equisetum* into the fire where their explosion in the heat was the treatment of the day. The din of their crackling and popping would jolt the languid tribesman from his lethargy, and send him on his way with new verve.

But the Horsetail was more than a trigger for vitality. Indians and settlers alike made a decoction of the barren limbs from which the pot-scouring substance, the silica, had been carefully stripped, and used it as a diuretic and an astringent. It was a favorite dropsy treatment; it was a potion reputed to encourage tardy menstruation; it was a common medicament for urinary ailments; applied externally, it was said to soothe wounds and cuts, stop their bleeding, and hasten the healing process.

Horsetail is still a popular herb today. Some modern herbalists claim it's beneficial for the hair, the skin, and the fingernails. Others suggest its use as a mouthwash, good for canker sores and other minor oral infections.

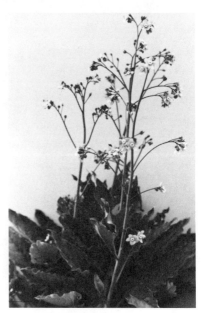

Hound's Tongue

HOUND'S TONGUE

Cynoglossum spp.

Other names for Hound's Tongue: Other popular English names were Blue Button, Coyote Ear, Dog Ear, Grand Hounds Tongue, and Burgundy Hounds Tongue. To the Yuki the plant was *Kochk.* To the Potter Valley Indians it was *De-wish-a-ma.*

Where to find it: In the early springtime Grand Hound's Tongue, *Cynoglossum grande,* a heavy-rooted native perennial plant, is a conspicuous early bloomer in its favorite haunts: half-shady woodlands, coast ranges, hillside forests, and dry slopes below 4,000 feet. The Burgundy Hounds tongue, *Cynoglossum officianale,* an alien biennial introduced from Eurasia, is found naturalized in northern Shasta County, six miles south of McCloud, in some Siskiyou County locations, and near Lake Arrowhead in southern California. Like the native Hounds Tongue, this plant is fond of shady spots, but prefers altitudes higher than the former would ever tolerate.

How to know it when you see it: Because of the shape and size of their long tapering leaves, which grow up to seven inches in length, these members of the forget-me-not family are often mistaken for Comfrey or Mullein. Their leaves are not as hairy as Mullein's or as coarse as Comfrey's, but they are similar enough that errors in identification are not surprising. Grand Hounds Tongue has large five-petaled flowers of clear bright blue, each of which bears an inner row of white teeth. The reddish-purple flowers of Burgundy Hounds Tongue, though similarly shaped and therefore best described as wheel-like, are nodding, and thickly arranged on sprays that appear to bend from their weight.

These flowers bear nutlike seeds, covered with little barbs that are like anchors when it comes to their ability to attach themselves to the hair of animals who pass in their vicinity. Thus they're distributed, and the Hounds Tongue is transported to another likely habitat.

Its lore. The native Hounds Tongue was probably a reputable medicinal plant of the California Indians long before there was anyone else around to observe its usage and try it out. The Concows applied the grated roots externally to burns and scalds and other injuries to soothe them and help them heal, while the natives of Potter Valley found these same roots a boon to common pains like stomach-aches. After the coming of the white man, whose advent brought so many maladies, some California tribes used this much-prized plant in the treatment of venereal diseases.

A late comer to California, the Burgundy Hounds Tongue also has a history as a highly-valued medicinal plant. In the Old World, not only was it used to treat diarrhea, coughs, and shortness of breath, it was considered a sedative and a narcotic, and even a good luck charm of a sort. According to an age-old legend, if an individual placed a Hounds Tongue leaf under his feet, whether bare or shod, he'd not be plagued by barking dogs. The hapless canine's tongue, it's said, would be firmly tied.

Today, in certain mountainous areas of the Southwest, where it's distribution is wider, Burgundy Hounds Tongue is used to make a fine root tea for dry coughs and sore throats, and a soothing decoction for hemorrhoids and piles.

INDIAN FIG

Opuntia megacantha and *O. Ficus-indica*

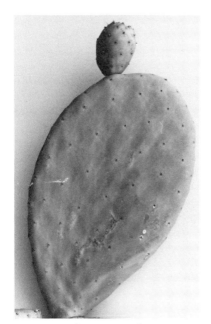

Indian Fig

Other names for the Indian Fig: Another popular name for Indian Fig was Tuna. The Cahuilla Indian called this plant *Navet*.

Where to find it: Once widely cultivated in California gardens, *Opuntia megacantha*, a native of the tropical Americas, still persists on its own, neglected and untended, here and there in various sections of the state. The same holds true for its similar relative, *O. Ficus-indica*. Despite their long residency in the states, these plants have been very slow to naturalize. Though not nearly as popular as they were when they were commonly regarded as a food and a medicine, they're still a familiar sight in gardens, and are, in fact, found there much more often than elsewhere.

How to know it when you see it: Familiar tree-like cacti with flat-jointed stems, these two species are much easier to identify than they are to handle or harvest—a feat best accomplished with caution and thick leather gloves. Their big fleshy joints are flat and oval—like Ping-pong paddles that have sprouted spines. In May and June these "paddles" sprout incredibly lovely flowers that are as wax-like in appearance as if they'd been carved from blocks of paraffin. Those of *O. megacantha* range in color from goldfinch yellow to yellowish-orange, whereas the blooms of its similar relative (the true Indian Fig) run from shades of gold to carnelian red. Later in the season these springtime wonders develop into the delicious purple fruit once so highly prized by the early Californios.

Its lore. It was the Spanish missionaries who brought this most versatile plant to California with them and cultivated it, sometimes in great hedgerows, in the wonderful mission gardens so often praised by the early visitors who saw them. Although he viewed them in the 1840s when they were already falling into disrepair, the roving journalist, Edwin Bryant, was clearly impressed by the plantings he saw at Mission San Luis Obispo. "There are several large gardens, enclosed by high and substantial walls," he wrote, "which now contain a great variety of fruit-trees and shrubbery. I noticed the orange, fig, palm, olive, and grape." It was here too that he became acquainted with the Indian Fig or Tuna plant, which he called "Prickly-Pear," but described in such a way that there can be little question concerning its identity. As he saw it, there were "large enclosures hedged in by the Prickly-Pear (cactus), which grows to an enormous size and makes an impervious barrier against man or beast. The stalks of some of these plants are of the thickness of a man's body, and grow to the height of fifteen feet. A juicy fruit is produced by the prickly-pear, named *tuna,* from which a beverage is sometimes made called *calinche.* It has a pleasant flavor, as has also the fruit, which, when ripe, is blood-red."

For many decades these mission gardens were the showplaces of the land, the storehouses of all good things to eat, and the "medicine factories" of the far west from which an assortment of remedies came pouring forth. In a sense they were comparable to the old European "physic gardens" of the sixteenth century, the property of apothecaries and physicians bent on following advice they'd gotten from *The Book Of Compounds.* In that great tome, a kind of handbook for healers, they were told that the garden of every apothecary "must be at hand, with plenty of herbs, seeds and roots to sow, set, plant, gather, preserve and keep." Those old-country gardens never featured Indian Fig, however, whereas on the mission grounds on the western edge of the new world, this plant was often the most conspicuous of all.

Indian Fig was truly a plant of many uses, affording fine healthful food, a thirst-quenching juice in times of emergency, a bandage for wounds, a poultice for sores, a compress for aches and pains, and even mortar for masonry!

Both the Spaniards and the Indians savored the fine purple fruit, which was often eaten raw but sometimes boiled and made into a syrup, sometimes further reduced into a kind of paste, a dark red substance called Qaueso de Tuna. But this much-favored food was "good medicine," too; it was supposed to reduce fevers, increase the flow of urine, cure pleurisy, treat mental disorders, take away chills, stop diarrhea, relieve an attack of asthma, and battle gonorrhea.

But as versatile as it was, this pride of early California had more to offer than its enticing fruit. There was a great demand for the pads as well. The young joints were gathered before the spines had hardened, cut into strips, and served as a potherb or made into pickles. When a water supply was depleted or tainted, their mucilaginous juice served as a good emergency drinking water, bitter-tasting but salvific nonetheless. Left whole, despined, split, and soaked in water, they were used—not only by the Indians and Spaniards but also by many a trapper, mountain man, prospector, and later-day settler—as a healing binding for cuts, bruises, dog bites, and insect stings. Heated to lukewarm, they were applied to the breasts of new mothers, where they were believed to ease soreness and help increase the supply of milk. Roasted over campfires, they were applied to the swollen faces of mumps victims, or the limbs and digits of those who suffered from gout. Cut into small bits, they served as healing "plugs" for the wounds of the Cahuilla. Mashed to a pulp, the joints made a good poultice for the stubborn sores of both humankind and animals, for arthritic swelling, and every kind of ache or pain.

In the old days, this plant was so valuable that no part of it went unused. Boiled in water, its stems made a good wash for curing headaches, soothing sore eyes, easing away the pains of rheumatism, and promoting sleep in insomniacs. The flowers went to make a tincture often suggested for disorders of the spleen. Even its fuzz wasn't wasted, but rather was used as a wart medicine, a remedy that was said not only to remove the unwelcome protuberance but to insure that it would never grow back again.

INDIAN HEMP

Apocynum spp.

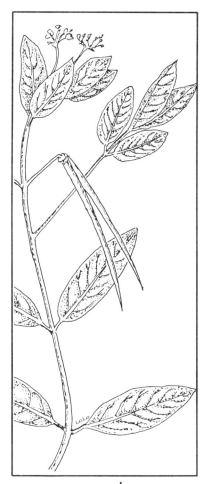

Indian Hemp

Other names for the Indian Hemp: Other popular English names for this plant are Dogbane, Black Hemp, Hemp Dogbane, Spreading Dogbane, Canadian Hemp, and Indian Silk. The Little Lake Indians called the Indian Hemp plant *Ma-sha*. To the Yokia it was *Si-lim ma*. To the Yuki it was *Ma*, and to the Concow, *Po*. The Spanish name for this old medicinal plant is *Lechuguila*.

Where to find it: One species of this genus, *A. cannabinum*, grows along ditches and in other moist waste places, at altitudes below 4,000 feet through most of California. *A. androsaemifolium*, however, which thrives in wilderness areas, on dry flats and slopes, and waste places, is found at altitudes up to to 9,500 feet.

How to know it when you see it: The leaves of Indian Hemp, which are wide-spaced and oval or lanceolate in shape, turn reddish-colored in the summer, as do its stems which are thin and round. The pale pink, terminal flowers of *A. androsaemifolium* appear in slightly drooping clusters, as do its leaves. The flowers of *A. cannabinum*, which is sometimes called Canadian Hemp, are a much less showy greenish-white; its leaves are rounder, and neither leaf nor flower possesses the drooping attitude that lends *A. androsaemifolium* some of its charm.

Its lore. For hundreds of years many California Indians cherished *A. cannabinum* most for the wonderfully utilitarian fiber that they collected, in the fall, from the inner bark of the plant. From this strong, silky material they produced their remarkably durable twine, nets, thread, ropes, and even some of the clothing they wore. Indian Hemp was such a valuable commodity for this reason, and prized so much because of it, that its uses as a remedy were distinctly secondary. Perhaps this was just as well, for its mountain-loving kin, *A. androsaemifolium*, is actually the safer of the two herbs (notably, both can be highly toxic to animals) and the one traditionally most often employed for medicinal purposes. It has been used as a cardiac tonic, as a diuretic, and as a treatment for alcoholism. It's such a potentially dangerous herb, however, that it's best left alone, except, perhaps, by those who'd like to try a unique treatment for hair loss. A brew of one teaspoon of the root of the Indian Hemp, boiled in a cup of water, cooled, and applied as a rinse to be poured on after shampooing, is said to mildly irritate the hair follicles and thereby stimulate growth.

Warning: Potentially, Indian Hemp (Dogbane) is extremely dangerous. Don't experiment with internal preparations. Leave further research to the ethnopharmacologists.

INDIAN MILKWEED

Asclepias eriocarpa

Other names for Indian Milkweed: The Concow called this plant *Bo-ko*. To the Little Lake it was *Go-to-la;* to the Yuki it was both *Ma-chal* and *Ch'a-ak*. To the Cahuilla it was *Kivat* or *Kiyal*.

Where to find it: Especially common from Mendocino and Shasta Counties southward, this woolly-leaved Milkweed thrives most in dry fields and other barren places below 7,000 feet.

How to know it when you see it: The sweet-scented, bee-beloved flowers of this big, conspicuous Milkweed are cream-colored, sometimes touched with a tint of pale purple. The woolly lance-shaped leaves are borne in whorls of three and four, occasionally in opposite pairs. It's this whorled arrangement and the marked width of the leaves that distinguish this plant from its kin, the Narrow-leaved Milkweed, and render it quite easy to identify.

Its lore. There are many species of Milkweed in California, and several of them have been used medicinally, first by the Indians, then by the Spaniards and latter-day settlers, and more recently by herbalists, survivalists, and wild-medicinal-plant enthusiasts all over the state. *A. asperula*, sometimes called by the name of "Immortal," is touted as a medicine for asthma, pleurisy, bronchitis, and an assortment of infections. *A. speciosa* is said to stimulate perspiration, increase the flow of urine, and encourage expectoration. *A. tuberosa*, better known as Butterfly Milkweed, is touted as a pleurisy remedy. *A. eriocarpa*, however, was apparently valued most by many Indians as an external medicine, an application for cuts, scratches, insect bites, and sores. It was used accordingly by all of the Round Valley Indian tribes except for the Yukis, who scorned it as a white man's remedy: testimony to the fact that the settlers must have used the herb in much the same way. It was the milky, gummy exudation of its leaves and stems that served as a lotion, a popular medicament reputed to heal and to soothe all kinds of minor cuts, sores, and scratches. Oddly enough, this was the selfsame substance that caused dermatitis in some individuals, burned off the warts of others, and poisoned the sheep who ate it, bringing on their agonizing death in less than half an hour.

INDIAN TOBACCO

Nicotiana bigelovii and other *Nicotiana* species

Other names for Indian Tobacco: *Nicotiana trigonophylla* is called Desert Tobacco. *N. attenuata* is best known as Coyote Tobacco. Another species, introduced from Peru, *N. glauca*, is referred to as Tree Tobacco. *N. bigelovii* is actually the true Indian Tobacco, but all of these species are sometimes referred to by that name. The Southern California Shoshonean Indians called tobacco *Pr pivat* or *Vs pibat*. To the Yokia it was *Sa-ka*.

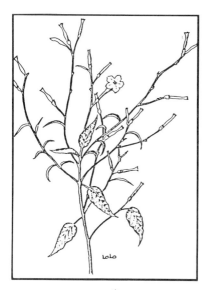

Indian Tobacco

Where to find it: Indian Tobacco is found growing in washes, on dryish plains and mesas, and in open valleys below 3,500 feet. Desert Tobacco, which thrives in the Mojave and Colorado Deserts, is often found growing around rocks in Creosote Bush scrub and Joshua Tree woods. Tree Tobacco flourishes in waste places, dry stream beds and arroyos in foothill areas at altitudes seldom exceeding 4,000 feet, while Coyote Tobacco seeks disturbed places in the Great Basin and in northern California, sometimes taking up in residential areas as well.

How to know it when you see it: Rarely does anyone describe these members of the Nightshade family in glowing terms. In his turn-of-the-century writings about the Indians' usage of plants that grew in Round Valley, V. K. Chestnut referred to *A. bigelovii* as "a very viscid and ill-smelling species of tobacco which is native to California and grows quite commonly along the dry beds of streams near Ukiah." Elsewhere, at the hand of a modern plant expert, the same plant is described as "dirty looking," while the non-native, Tree Tobacco, is referred to as "scraggly" and "unkempt" and as bearing flowers of a "sickly" shade of yellow. Even in the non-judgmental and objective terms of a popular field guide, *N. attenuata* is "bad-smelling."

A "touch test" is helpful too in identifying this much-maligned plant. It's foliage feels distinctly wet and sticky, like a dishcloth that's just been used to wipe up a blob of spilled syrup. With clues like these, and a word or two about the flowers of *nicotiana*, it shouldn't be too difficult to identify the well known wild tobaccos that flourish in California. The blooms in question are generally trumpet-shaped and would be quite lovely if one could divorce them from the rest of the plant, from its smell, its stickiness, and its spindly form. Those of *N. trigonophylla* are greenish-white; those of *N. attenuata* the aforementioned "sickly yellow."

Its lore. California Indians generally had more reasons than sociability or hedonism to smoke their nicotine. This is not to say that smoking for pleasure was alien to all tribes (though it was indeed to some, the Karoks, for example). To certain tribes of California Indians, a spirit of camaraderie was truly a vital part of the evening smoking sessions. But the point is that sociability and pleasure were not the *only* motivation for their use of this poisonous and narcotic plant.

Although it may not seem so on the surface, this is probably even true when it comes to a particular practice of the Channel Islands Indians, whose nicotine habits were certainly unique. From two simple ingredients, common Wild Tobacco and pulverized seashells, they prepared a pasty substance called *peribate,* a mixture made for chewing, which left them highly intoxicated only moments after they'd mouthed it. According to records, they much preferred this concoction to the white man's beloved brandy.

To the California tribesmen (even, no doubt, to those innovative Channel Island natives) tobacco was an admirable and respected plant, the use of which was almost sacrosanct. How could it have been otherwise? Wasn't it an important herb of the shamans—they who knew how to enact cures by blowing its smoke upon their patients in a certain healing manner? Wasn't it greatly favored by legendary folk heros like the Yurok's powerful Pulekukwerek, who knew how the sky was woven and who'd put the stars in place, a benefactor of mankind who smoked but never ate, and who knew how to kill monsters and evil people with the same plant he smoked himself? And what of the Cahuilla legend in which Tobacco was one of the first plants created by the great god, Mukat. Straight from his heart, he drew both the plant and a pipe with which to smoke it.

With the shamans of many tribes, Tobacco smoking—prayerfully done, of course—constituted a means of diagnosing illnesses. And some tribes, especially the Yurok, the Yahi, and the Yokuts, used the much-valued plant as a religious offering. To the Luisenos the herb was a substance with which a young girl just entering womanhood could prove her worth. If she didn't vomit the balls of Tobacco she was made to swallow, if somehow she managed to hold them down, she was considered virtuous indeed.

Among the tribes of the lower Klamath area, nicotine smoking was almost a cult. With the Karoks it was a ritual and a rite with a definite end, part of a tribal custom. And even those Indians who did indeed smoke for pleasure were often doing so simultaneously for religious or medicinal purposes. Smoking was widely believed to calm the nerves, to soothe the worried mind, to cure colds, and to promote sleep. And when Tobacco was mixed with Desert sage, Cough root, or Indian balsam, and the whole concoction smoked, it was believed good for asthma, for stubborn coughs, and even for tuberculosis.

Most Indians were as fond of the white man's cultivated tobacco as they were of the wild-growing varieties. As Bryant learned from experience, any friendly encounter between native and newcomer was apt to involve some exchange of this favored substance. Of such a meeting in Bear Valley, he wrote: "One of the half-breeds, of a pleasing and intelligent countenance and good address, introduced us to their chief (El Capitan), and wished to know if we had not some tobacco to give him, I had a small quantity of tobacco about half of which I gave to the chief, and distributed the residue among the party as far as it would go. I saw, however, that the chief divided his portion among those who received none."

Some tribes, the Yurok, for one, scorned the use of any Tobacco that grew in the wild. What if it had sprouted forth from a gravesite, or from seed that had been produced on a grave? The wilding did have a predilection for just such sites, and no one could argue it. Wasn't such contamination too hazardous to risk? Wasn't it safer to cultivate the plant rather than to pick it in the wild? It was from just such reasoning that this northern tribe, these non-agricultural Yuroks, engaged in this totally uncharacteristic behavior: they farmed. It's true their pursuits went no further than the burned-off plots of ground on which they nursed their crops of *nicotiana* (the very same species that grew wild all around them and was theirs for the picking if they only dared), but it was agriculture nonetheless, however small the scale. Unlikely as it sounds, the Yuroks were California's first Tobacco farmers.

Whether cultivated or not, *nicotiana* had a number of popular medicinal uses. As a steamed-leaf poultice it was a pain-killer for earache and toothache, for rheumatism, edema, eczema, for cuts, and rattlesnake bites. Even the settlers, those from the states and those from Europe, sometimes turned to this homely plant for relief from their ills. It was not surprising that they did; they may have been abiding by the herbalists of the era, especially those who swore by the methods of that old plant wizard, Nicholas Culpeper. Significantly enough, at least two of his prescribed usages for another species of the plant, *nicotiana tabacum* (a cure for rheumatism, and a treatment for toothache) were the same as those that the early Californians employed for their scraggly wild Tobaccos. He also suggested an ointment made of Tobacco leaves and hog's lard to be used for painful piles; a decoction of powdered leaves as a louse repellent; and the smoke of the herb administered as a clyster to revive individuals who'd nearly drowned.

In point of fact, poisonous as it is, Tobacco boasts a rich tradition of medicinal use.

JIMSON WEED

Datura spp.

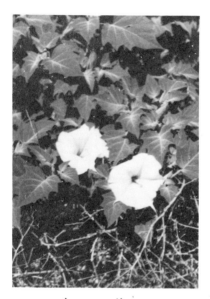

Jimson Weed

Other names for Jimson Weed: Other common English names for Jimson Weed are Datura, Sacred Datura, Mad Apple, Thorn Apple, Devil's Apple, and Devil Weed. The Yokut Indians called this herb *Tanai*. To the Cahuillas it was *Kiksaw-va'al*. Spanish Californios called this plant *Toloache*, a word which comes directly from the Aztec.

Where to find it: This historic and potentially lethal wild plant is found growing, usually in large stands, in sandy or gravelly soil. Expect to find it in the Mojave and Colorado Deserts, in Joshua Tree woods, in Creosote Bush scrub, along the coast, in foothills and on dry mountains, by ditches, and on shoulders of backroads and highways, washes, and gullies.

How to know it when you see it: Ironically, this lover of parched places looks like an escapee from some mythical rain forest where each plant is pregnant with the darkest of secrets—and will bear them tomorrow like great showy flowers. Although it differs from species to species, generally Jimson Weed is an herb of large proportions, clumped upon its gravelly bed like a gargantuan bouquet, multi-branched, with stems that seem to be made of rubber, broad green leaves like construction-paper cutouts, and a rank smell that's heavily unpleasant. It's rarely perceived as a pretty plant. Sometimes it's so insect-infested that its great floppy leaves are riddled with holes, but the Jimson Weed does indeed have showy flowers. Sometimes white, sometimes an almost luminous pale lavender, occasionally purple, these great blooms are as trumpet-like as Morning Glories and oftentimes even more beautiful.

Its lore. The most important thing to realize about Jimson Weed, a fact always well-known to the Indians who used it, is that this is a dangerous plant, a deadly drug, and it must be handled with respect and fear and never regarded lightly.

It's true that some of the native Californians, the Cahuilla Indians, for example, actually smoked or drank this deadly poison more than once in a lifetime, as at ceremonial dances or before important hunting treks. For most Indians, however, the use of Jimson Weed marked a once-in-a-lifetime occasion, a sacramental event, a time for prayer and meditation. (Among tribes that used Jim-

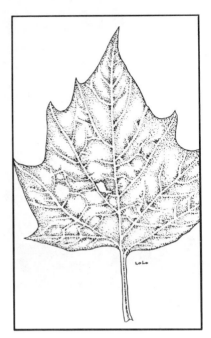

Jimson Weed

son Weed were the aforementioned Cahuilla, the Gabrielino, the Luiseno, the Diegueno, the Chumash, the Dumna, and the Yokuts.)

For the special occasion of its consumption, these early Californians made a strong potion of the herb's potent roots and drank it down, knowing full well that it would make them dreadfully delirious; that the visions it would give them would fill them with fear; that they'd fall into a stupor; that they might vomit; they might die; that if they didn't die they might well wish they could. Paradoxically, they believed that Jimson Weed and the initiation ceremonies attending its use could cure their ills, prepare them for adulthood, strengthen them physically, uplift them morally, enrich them spiritually, and even ensure their future domestic and economic success. Nevertheless, they never downed that all-important draught until they were properly schooled and spiritually prepared, until they'd fasted for days, and prayed for hours, and until they were carefully guided on their hazardous trip into the occult by some individual of profound wisdom and a world of experience.

To these tribes who prized *Toloache*, the herb was far more than a medicinal plant. It was sacrosanct. It's fair to say that the plant and its ceremony could actually be considered a religion. It was at once the cult and the sacrament of the cult; it was both a reason to pray and a prayer itself.

Although the benefits derived from the ceremonial consumption of the herb were believed to be long-term, perhaps even lifelong, the *Toloache* rite was usually a one-time event, primarily a puberty rite, an initiation into the world of adults, in which most of the initiates were youngsters ranging in age from twelve to fifteen. There were exceptions, however. Some individual members of the Jimson Weed cult took part in the ceremony more than once in their youth. Others passed through their puberty without ever having imbibed the drug at all. Sometimes, as in the case of one particular old southern Yokut, it was never consumed until a time came when a physical condition was to demand its medicinal use. According to his story, he was well into his manhood when he broke his arm and treated the injury by consuming a Jimson Root decoction on twelve alternate nights, remaining in a stupor all the while.

Of course, members of the Jimson Weed cult used this powerful herb for many ailments besides broken bones. The crushed plant was applied as a poultice not only to minor injuries like common bruises and swellings, but severe trauma too: the bites of tarantulas and rattlesnakes. Sometimes, as in cases when ailing animals were particularly valuable or especially beloved, a Jimson Weed compress was even applied to sores on horses.

It's interesting to note that Indians of tribes that did *not* follow the Jimson Weed cult generally did not take the drug orally. Many never used it in any way at all. Apparently early Californians realized that this herb was far too dangerous to be consumed by those who did not consider it holy.

This is not to say that only the Indians belonging to the Jimson Weed cult have ever used the herb medicinally. Applied externally, it was a useful medicament of many an early settler. In the form of smoke (from a small sprinkling of dried leaves tossed upon a fire), it's long been considered a reputable treatment for asthma attacks. Even today some survivalists tout it as a fresh-herb poultice for pains of arthritis or neuralgia. But anyone (except members of the Jimson Weed cult) who has ever been so foolish as to take this drug orally has lived to regret it, if they've lived at all.

The author still shudders at the recollection of a young man she saw once in the intensive care unit of a community hospital, a thrill-seeker who had decided to experiment with this highly hallucinatory herb. Spread-eagled in a bed, tightly bound so as to keep him from doing physical damage to himself or others, he was near death. He was terribly tormented, screaming aloud at whatever demons were plaguing him, begging for help. Whether he lived or died I do not know. One thing is certain: if he did survive, he's certainly steered clear of Jimson Weed ever since.

Warning: The use of this plant may cause severe mental disorientation, extreme locomotor problems, dangerous cardiac symptoms, and other serious physical complications, with effects that range from psychosis to death. Ironically, it is human beings rather than livestock who have suffered most often from Jimson Weed poisoning. This is not to say that the latter never suffer such a fate; there is, in fact, a case on record in which several members of a flock of lambs in Stanislaus County died from having consumed *Datura*. Generally, however, the plant is so distasteful to animals that they take care to avoid it.

JOJOBA

Simmondsia chinensis

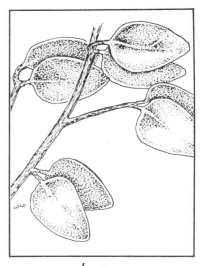

Jojoba

Other names for Jojoba: Two other common English names for *Simmondsia chinensis* are Goatnut and Deer Nut. To the Cahuilla Indians the plant was *Qawnaxal.*

Where to find it: Often found keeping company with plants like Mormon Tea, Bladder Sage, and the Desert Almond, this useful herb is a common denizen of desert washes and oases, dry barren slopes, Creosote brushland, Joshua Tree woods, and chaparral country, in southern California locations below 5,000 feet.

How to know it when you see it: This stiff-branched shrub grows to about seven feet in height, bears dense little flowers of greenish-yellow, and nut-like fruit that's acorn-shaped, brownish-black in color, and stuffed with a big oily seed that yields the substance for which this plant is so highly prized.

Jojoba exhibits an interesting way of withstanding the heat of the habitats where it grows; a feature which happens also to be one of its distinguishing earmarks. Its opposite and rather leathery leaves turn up toward the sun nowhere but at their edges.

Its lore. Jojoba was an important food of many southern tribes of Indians whose stark habitat it shared. The Cahuillas in particular greatly valued the rich oily nut. They consumed it just as it was and also used it to make a nutritious and refreshing beverage, much savored by the youngsters of the tribe.

Settlers appreciated this plant too and were quick to learn that it afforded a fine emollient, a hair tonic, a shampoo ingredient and replenishing oil, more effective, it seemed, than anything they'd found in the stores back home. Naturally then, it wasn't long until Jojoba itself was to hit the shelves, in the form of the whole nuts which were sold in early Los Angeles drug stores as a hair restorer, a scalp conditioner, and an eyebrow oil.

Recently, since Jojoba has been recognized as a good substitute for sperm-whale oil, interest in its commercial cultivation has dramatically risen. Once again its a "store bought" commodity, Jojoba shampoos, tonics, oils, and creams, and even a few pharmaceutical preparations can be found here and there on drugstore shelves. This is poetic justice in the eyes of modern herbalists who often look to yesterday to see what may be useful now and tomorrow and a century from now.

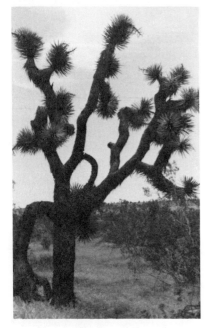

Joshua Tree

JOSHUA TREE

Yucca brevifolia

Other names for the Joshua Tree: Other English names for this remarkable desert dweller are Yucca, Tree Yucca, and Soap Tree. To the Cahuilla Indians the plant was known as was *Humwichawa*.

Where to find it: One sure place to find this unusual tree is, of course, in the park that bears its name, the picturesque Joshua Tree National Monument in Southern California. There, the weird form in all its wild variations is as familiar a sight as the desert sky against which it is so dramatically silhouetted. But so it is elsewhere too, as in wide areas of the Mojave Desert and in Owens Valley, and on dry mesas and slopes in other arid Southern California locations as well.

How to know it when you see it: Growing sometimes to a height of thirty feet, the very photogenic Joshua Tree often looms high above the other desert plants with which it keeps company. Its stiff, blue-green leaves, forming in clusters at the ends of the multi-shaped branches, range from six to ten inches in length, are pointed at the tips, and finely toothed. Its creamy-white flowers (which only bloom when temperatures and rainfall are especially propitious) appear in thick clusters about a foot in length.

Its lore. Like those of its relative, Our Lord's Candle (*Yucca baccata*), and other Yuccas, the roots of this impressive resident of the California desert once provided a dependable cleanser to the land's early residents. Considered a good all-purpose soap, it was used for washing a variety of household items, not to mention hands and faces and hair. For imparting sheen to the latter, some claimed it could vie with Jojoba; as a dandruff treatment it was on par with Amole. But these cosmetic usages were trivial when compared to some of the others the Joshua Tree had to its credit. In the form of a good strong infusion made from the same roots that rid the scalp of pesky dandruff, it was once a popular treatment for the venereal diseases that the white man had brought.

JUNIPER

Juniperus spp.

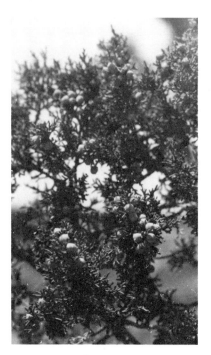

Juniper

Other names for the Juniper: Other popular English names for the Juniper are Cedar and Incense Cedar. To the Yokia Indians the plant was *Spo ka-la*. The Cahuilla called it *Yuyily*. The Spanish name for Juniper is *Sabina*.

Where to find it: From the scrubby little Utah Juniper to its taller Rocky Mountain kin, most Junipers thrive on hillsides and slopes in dry rocky soil. You'll find one species of *Juniperus* or another in the company of such plants as the Joshua Tree, Flannel Bush, the California Poppy and Mexican Manzanita.

How to know it when you see it: Depending on species and habitat, *Juniperus* varies considerably in size and shape. Roughly speaking, there are two types: those that are tree-sized, scaly-twigged and leafless; and those that are shrubsized, spreading and needled. The Rocky Mountain Juniper grows to a height of 40 feet, whereas its kin, the Utah Juniper, is only half that size. But the bark of all species as well as the berry, the leaf, or the twig, is highly aromatic. Green when young, whitewashed purplish-blue when ripe, the berries smell very much like the gin that's their derivative. If you're in doubt as to the identity of the small tree or shrub you're studying, then pick one of its fruits, pierce its flesh with your thumbnail, put it up to your nose, close your eyes and whiff. If you catch the unmistakable "ginny" scent , you've found that tried old westerner, that medicine of many early-day Californians known as the Juniper.

Its lore. In the folk medicine of the American west the Juniper ranked high on the list of versatile cure-alls. Indians made use of every single part of the plant from its fibrous bark, used to make diapers for infants, to its stems which were mashed to make poultices and plasters for toothaches and stiff joints. Berries were brewed to make an infusion applied to aching parts of rheumatism victims. Steam from smoldering wet juniper branches was an inhalant. The branches themselves, placed over the glowing embers of a dying campfire, served as a steaming "bed" upon which the aching patient, bundled in blankets, would recline and await the easing of pain. Berries and twigs were eaten by warriors readying themselves for battle. Warm mashed-berry plasters were applied to sprained ankles and swollen knees or bound over burns, scratches, scalds, and cuts. Pulverized dried twigs were sprinkled over slow-to-heal sores. Juniper berries carried in a pocket or a "medicine bundle" warded away evil spirits and promoted good fortune. The smoke from Juniper leaves was used to fumigate sick rooms. A concoction of warmed Juniper resin and ripe berries served as a drawing salve for boils and skin infections. And the panacea of panaceas, Juniper Berry tea, was administered to strengthen and invigorate, to combat internal hemorrhaging, to correct uterine obstructions, to treat assorted kidney ailments, to cure colds and sore throats, to treat urinary tract infections, to serve as a birth control medicine, to ease gassy stomach, to expel worms, to counteract constipation, relieve hiccups, treat hardening of the arteries, and to deal with dreaded snakebite.

Many early settlers, especially those still abiding by the old-country herbalists, were just as enthusiastic about the Juniper as the Indians were. These individuals believed that this plant could strengthen their brains, improve their eyesight, break up kidney stones, and fight the plague. They'd not have been without a stock of the beneficent little purple berries in their larders. Neither, for that matter, would many a modern herbalist, for Juniper is one of the old medicinals that has really never fallen from favor. It's true, of course, that it may no longer be touted as a brain strengthener or a pestilence cure, but it is still used as a diuretic and an antiseptic, as a carminative, as a delightful culinary herb, and as a featured scent of those aroma therapists who feel that a fresh woodland fragrance can help to ease a case of high-tech stress.

Warning: Overconsumption of berries, or heavy and/or extended inhalation of any parts of the Juniper, or even more moderate inhalation by sensitive individuals, can cause nausea, stomach upset, dermatitis, and other complications. Pregnant women should avoid this plant entirely.

LACEPOD

Thysanocarpus curvipes

Other names for the Larkspur: This plant is called Delphinium almost as often as it's called Larkspur. The Calpella Indians called it *So-ma-yem*. To an English-speaking Yuki it was "Lady's Slipper."

Where to find it: A common plant, Lacepod thrives in dry or sandy soil mostly below 5,000 feet. It's found on grassy or brushy slopes, amidst coastal sage scrub, in chaparral, and in woodsy foothills in many California locations.

How to know it when you see it: There's considerable variation between one Lacepod plant and another, but generally speaking, this is a slender herb, twelve to eighteen inches high, with coarsely-toothed, oblong basal leaves, small stem leaves, and inconspicuous white flowers. But it's the markedly pendulous seed pods that develop from those modest flowers that are its most distinguishing feature. Like miniature versions of those round linen doilies so popular in the nineteenth century, they're about a quarter of an inch in diameter and bear around their edges a fringe that truly does resemble fine tatted lace.

Its lore. Beyond the fact that at least two tribes of California Indians made a tea from the whole Lacepod plant to be used as a treatment for stomach-ache, and a tea of the leaves alone for colic, little is known about this old medicinal plant.

LARKSPUR

Delphinium spp.

Other names for the Larkspur: This plant is called *Delphinium* almost as often as it's called Larkspur. The Calpella Indians called it *So-ma-yem*. To an English-speaking Yuki it was "Lady's Slipper."

Where to find it: There are so many species of this poisonous plant flourishing within the state that it wouldn't do to name more than just a few. Generally speaking the tall Larkspurs, some of which reach a height of five or six feet, prefer moist habitats and comparatively high elevation, while their shorter relatives, rarely exceeding two feet in height, lean toward grassy fields, foothills, valleys, and even deserts.

Perhaps the most destructive of all California's Larkspurs, since it grows in such wild profusion, is *Delphinium menziesii,* which is found in open places near the ocean, especially in Mendocino County. *D. nudicaule,* a species familiar to the Calpella and Yuki tribes, is found on dry slopes, and among shrubs in wooded areas, mostly in the northern part of the state at altitudes up to 6,500 feet. *D. hesperium,* another northerner, is found on grassy slopes and ridges, in foothill woods, and on inner coast ranges at altitudes below 3,000 feet. *D. parishii* thrives on gravelly benches and washes, in Creosote Bush scrub, Joshua Tree woods, and amidst Pinyons and Junipers in Southern California at altitudes below 7,500 feet. *D. parryi* is common on open slopes and mesas, in grassland, in coastal sage scrub, chaparral, Oak woods and Pine forests, at altitudes below 6,500 feet. *D. cardinale,* the lovely Scarlet Larkspur, populates openings in woods and brushland from Monterey County to San Diego County and on down into lower California.

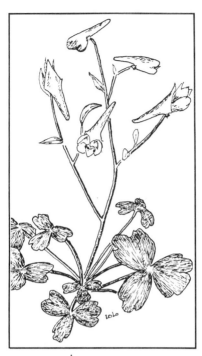

Larkspur

How to know it when you see it: Of the many species of Larkspur native to California (approximately thirty), most are erect and branching perennial herbs which bear their flowers in great showy spikes or racemes. Of those mentioned above, the flowers of *D. menziesii* are dark blue; those of *D. nudicaule* are reddish yellow; those of *D. hesperium* are dark blue or blue-purple with white-edged petals; those of *D. parryi,* purplish-blue, and those of *D. cardinale* a deep true red. Larkspur flowers each bear a distinctive backward-projecting spur that, happily enough, renders their identification a rather easy matter.

Its lore. To the tribes who knew it well, the Larkspur was apparently most notable for its narcotic properties. In fact, the literal meaning of *So-ma-yem,* the Calpella name for the Larkspur, is nothing other than "sleeproot," a word that would seem to indicate the herb may have been used as a remedy for insomnia. Records are silent on that use, yet audible when it comes to another—that of drugging an unsuspecting enemy in a game of chance. Apparently a gambler who'd been stupefied by a dose of Larkspur represented little threat to his cunning opponent.

But the Larkspurs of California are better known for another usage entirely. For well over a century, a tincture of Larkspur (one part of ground flowers steeped for a week in five parts of vinegar or rubbing alcohol) was the old standby treatment for cases of head lice, body lice, scabies, and other "varmints" and vexations.

Caution: This widespread and common plant—every species of which is highly toxic—is probably responsible for more cattle poisoning than any other group of plants in the state. Since *Delphinium* isn't normally consumed by human beings, the hazard here is small, except in the case of foolish experimentation by adults or accidental sampling by children. Symptoms of Larkspur poisoning include a burning sensation in the mouth, prickling sensation of skin, headache, low blood pressure, nervousness, nausea, depression, vomiting, weak pulse, and convulsions. Death may follow.

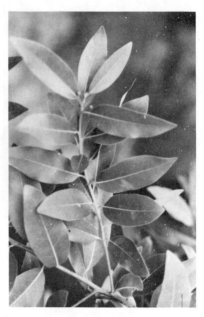

Laurel

LAUREL

Umbellularia californica

Other names for the Laurel Tree: English speaking Californians have called this tree California Bay, Oregon Myrtle, California Laurel, Pepperwood Tree, California Pepper Tree, Balm Of Heaven, Spice Bush, and Headache Tree. The Numlaki Indians called it *So-e-ba*. To the Pomo it was *Ba hem*; to the Concow *So-e-ba*. Its Yuki name was *Pol-cum ol*.

Where to find it: From San Diego on northward through the Sierra Nevadas, this handsome tree is found growing on all the western ranges, in canyons and damp woods, and by foothill streams, usually below 5,000 feet.

How to know it when you see it: The smooth-margined, lanceolate, evergreen leaves of the California Laurel are by far its most distinguishing feature. When crushed in the hand, their aroma, variously described as camphor-like, spicy, medicinal, and "kitcheny," is perceptible at once. It's a pleasing scent to most people, unpleasant to others, unforgettable in either case. Once it's smelled it's recognized immediately ever after. (Don't whiff it too long, however. Lengthy inhalation can invite a headache which is best treated, it's said, by a goodly dose of Laurel-leaf tea!)

The bark of this useful old medicinal tree is greenish-brown. Its small clustered flowers are yellow-green in color, its fruit purplish. Usually comparatively small, sometimes only shrub-sized, the Laurel does occasionally reach a height of 80 feet, in which case it's a handsome tree, slender-branched, well-shaped, pleasing to the eye of any woodland rover.

Its lore. To cure headaches or to rid the head of vermin early Californians would either poke Laurel leaves under their hats or bonnets, tie them to their foreheads with a sash or a strip of leather, or dab their heads with cloths that had been dipped in a good strong Laurel tea. For the headache, if not the vermin, they'd drink a cup of the same infusion and wait expectantly for the pain to recede. As a counterirritant for stomach problems, they'd bind themselves with strips of cloth, under which they'd poke a quantity of mashed or crumbled leaves, and wear it thusly for a day or two. For the pains of rheumatism they'd bathe in hot water in which the leaves had been steeped, or rub themselves with an ointment concocted of leaves and lard.

A Laurel leaf treatment said to be beneficial for many types of ailments, and one that often left the user as covered with smudge as a chimneysweep, required that the leaves be thrown upon a slow-burning fire, or upon its dying embers, and that the aromatic vapor be breathed until symptoms were relieved.

Laurel leaves were also reputedly an excellent insecticide (said to drive away even the heartiest of fleas when strewn about the yard), a good "smelling salt," and, administered as a tea, a fine cure for neuralgia and cramps and gastroenteritis.

Apparently the reputation of this aromatic old medicinal plant far transcended its own habitat, for in 1823 a Spaniard, who lived in Honolulu, wrote a letter to the Californio Don Luis Antonio Arguello in which he requested (among other things like shoe leather and chamois skins) some Laurel seeds that he might plant on those distant shores.

Even today, many herbalists look as kindly upon the aromatic *Umbellularia californica* as do the countless craftsmen who prize it not for its leaves but for its fine wood. (It's beautiful; it lends itself well to polish and lathe work; it's economically important.) As nineteenth-century Californians might well have foretold, its ever-potent greenery is still used today as an old stand-by pain reliever, a boon to the achy, the crabbed, and the cramped.

Comment: Contact with California Laurel leaves has been known to cause skin irritations in some individuals, headaches in others, and sneezing in a few. When used as a culinary spice, the dried leaves should be used more sparingly than those of the true bay leaf, *Laurus nobilis*.

LICORICE

Glycyrrhiza spp.

Other names for Licorice: Our native species, *G. lepidota*, is sometimes called American Licorice, Sweet Root, and Wild Licorice. The Spanish name for Licorice is *Amolillo*.

Where to find it: Sometimes found in rich, moist lowland areas near ditches and gullies and streams, Wild Licorice, *G. lepidota*, generally does best in middle mountain habitats at altitudes up to 7,500 feet. Even there, however, it seeks out streamsides, irrigation ditches, and other damp and sloped locations, much like those it favors at lower altitudes.

The more popular and much-used cultivated licorice, *G. glabra*, which hails from Eurasia, is an occasional escapee from gardens and dooryards, and is naturalized just enough to rate its place on these pages. It's found growing wild near Pomona and around Kern County's Goose Lake.

How to know it when you see it: The Wild Licorice plant, which rather resembles the sweet pea, grows in large colonies, connected one to the other by long creeping rootstalks, and reaches heights that range from one to four feet. Its leaflets, which are slightly sticky to the touch, are arranged in pairs along the stems until they reach the tips, where a single leaflet marks the end. Hence these little "lances" always contain an odd number of leaflets, ranging from eleven to seventeen. The plant bears oblong capsules covered with hooked hairs, and clover-like blossoms, white or pale yellowish-green in color, that stand erect in brushy heads.

G. glabra, which grows wild so profusely in the Mediterranean, so rarely in California, follows much the same description as its American relative. Its leaf-

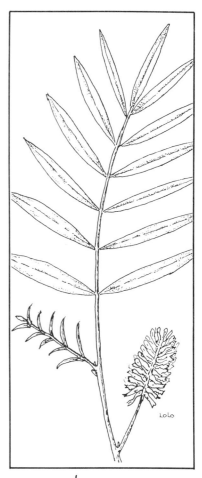

Licorice

lets are lance-shaped and odd-numbered and it too grows from long winding runners. *G. glabra*, however, boasts long-stemmed spikes of lovely bluish-purple or violet-blue flowers, much more showy than those of *G. lepidota*.

Its lore. Records indicate that the Wild Licorice plant may not have played as big a role in the folk medicine of the California Indians as it did in that of native Americans elsewhere—like the Sioux who used the root of the plant for their toothaches and drops of strong tea made from its leaves to ease their aching ears. Early settlers, however, reared as they were on Licorice decoctions, syrups, and tisanes, must have been delighted to find the plant growing wild in their new home, ready for them to pick and use in the manner of their ancestors—for coughs, for scratchy throats, for chest congestion, and for constipation.

Modern herbalists feel that either species of Licorice can serve as an excellent treatment for minor upper respiratory complications, for chronic menstrual cramps, and as a mild laxative.

Licorice has never truly lost its reputation. Even many modern pharmacologists believe it may be a worthwhile remedy for common coughs.

Comment: Pregnant women and persons with high blood pressure should avoid the use of this herb.

MADRONE

Arbutus menziesii

Other names for the Madrone: Other English names are Pacific Madrone and Madrona. The Yuki called this tree *Foin-ka*. To the Concows it was both *Dis-ta-tsi* and *kou-wat-chu*. The Little Lake name was *Ki-ya*, and the Yokia called it *Kab-it*. The Spanish name for this tree is *Madrono*.

Where to find it: Always seeming to favor woodsy slopes and rocky soil, often found in the company of Douglas Firs, Oaks, and Bays, this lovely tree with the ever-changing bark was once a common sight from British Columbia all the way down into lower California. Although it's still a familiar tree in some southern parts of the state (such as Ventura County, the San Gabriel Mountains, and near San Diego County's Mount Palomar), it's gradually losing much of its southern habitat and is now far more abundant in the northern parts of the state.

Sometimes the Madrone is a part of the understory in forests of taller trees, and there it stands, sharing filtered light and shadow-play with other trees such as Tanoaks, Laurels, and Giant Chinquapin.

How to know it when you see it: The Madrone is a tree with many features that endear it at once to the eye of the woodland rover. Its heavy branches yield so much shade it's easy to see how it offered such comfort to the old Indian villages, how the dark-eyed children would gather beneath it and play in its flickering shadows. It's stately; it's evergreen; its alternate leaves are thick and

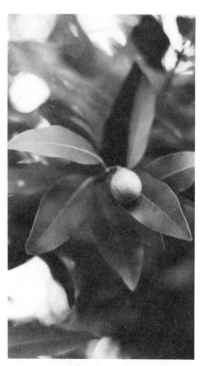

Madrone

glossy. Growing sometimes to a height of 100 feet, its crown is wide and spreading. In the month of May it's graced with clusters of creamy-white or vaguely pinkish flowers that are so bell-shaped one can almost fancy they're bound to ring. And later, at the waning of summer or the first flush of fall, it's covered with orangy-red berries, round and mealy, beloved to birds and other inveterate berry-pickers.

But as attractive as they are, none of these features of the handsome Madrone can vie with the one that happens to be its most distinguishing earmark: its fascinating, ever-changing bark. It's an exfoliating covering, this bark of *Arbutus menziesii*, and in early July it begins to fall away in thin, papery layers, in irregular sections, to uncover a surface that's pale greenish-brown at first but fades, at length, into a lovely sherry-wine color that truly feasts the eye. These exposed parts are incredibly smooth and look as if they've been painstakingly polished by some master craftsman.

Its lore. The Madrone was once a dependable medicinal plant to many California Indians and to those adaptable settlers who chose to follow suit. The Little Lake Indians brewed an infusion of the glossy leaves and used it to treat their colds. A similar leaf decoction served as a cure for stomach ailments of the Cahuilla. Others made a lotion of both leaves and bark with which they dabbed their own sores and cuts, as well as those of their beloved horses, to hasten healing.

Comment: Madrone berries are edible when either raw or dried, but as their consistency is mealy and their taste somewhat bitter, they're best eaten after adding sugar or honey and cooking into a sauce.

MALLOW

Malva spp.

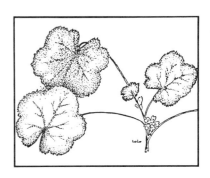

Mallow

Other names for Mallow: This plant is also known as Cheese Plant, Cheese Mallow, Cheeseweed, Umbrella Mallow, and Curled Mallow.

Where to find it: Natives of Eurasia, there are several species of *Malva* growing wild in California. *M. sylvestris*, commonly called High Mallow, is still considered only a garden escapee; *M. nicaeensis* is an occasional weed in waste places, and Curled Mallow, *M. verticillata*, is apparently naturalized only in the North Bay county of Marin. But *M. neglecta*, sometimes called Umbrella Mallow, and *M. parviflora*, best known as Cheeseweed, are practically ubiquitous. You'll find them in waste places all over the state.

How to know it when you see it: Since these relatives of the Hollyhock are at once a common weed and a rather innocuous one, they often go unnoticed. Then too, some species tend to hug the ground, a feature that renders them all the more inconspicuous. Sometimes, however, especially in rich moist places, even the lowly *M. neglecta* can reach up to a foot in height. High Mallow, *M. sylvestris*, apparently the favorite of early old-country herbalists, is much more apt to gain attention than any of its small-flowered kin. Not only is it taller, sometimes growing to a height of four feet, but it bears lovely dark-veined, purplish-rose blooms an inch in width. The leaves of most Mallows are markedly lobed, pointed in some species, rounded in others, and number from five to seven, depending on the species.

Its lore. When the great "natural philosopher" Jose Longinos Martinez made his expedition to California in 1792, this foreign plant was already thriving in the new land. According to his commentary, "the common apothecary's Mallow, which was not known in those countries, has been propagated from some seeds which were sent mixed with others—so much so that it is very difficult each year to clear it out. It grows with such vigor that because of it, one cannot walk in the immediate vicinity of the missions or through certain grainfields." The innovative padres of Mission San Diego had actually "manufactured several hundredweight of it to see if some profit may not be had from it," and had discovered, in the process that a fine yarn could be made from the carded Mallow fiber, and that it was of such quality that it "could be used for any cloth suitable for the clothing of the Indians . . ."

Martinez didn't mention the medicinal uses to which the padres put this hearty plant, but surely *Malva* was employed in California just as it had been in the old country: primarily as a soothing herb for ailments of the urinary tract, administered sometimes as a strong root decoction, sometimes as a flower conserve, sometimes in a mixture with a syrup of violets.

Mallow had other medicinal uses too, of course. Through the years it's been used variously as a treatment for digestive disturbances, for coughs and colds, for upper respiratory problems, for intestinal complaints, and as an ingredient in many a poultice, applied (usually in a warm pasty mass) to stings, bites, swellings, ulcers and sores of every type.

Mallow is one of those herbs that has managed somehow to hold its own. Even weed experts and pharmacologists tend to view it with a certain tolerance and many modern herbalists, some of whom claim that the roots of *Malva* tastes like Ginseng, warmly tout it as a fine demulcent and emollient, effective in lessening pain and soothing inflammation.

MANZANITA

Arctostaphylos manzanita

Other names for the Manzanita: Other common English names for the Manzanita are Little Apple, Mealy Plum, and Mealberry. To the Cahuilla Indians Manzanita was *Kelel*. The Numlaki Indians called it *Pa-got*. The Yuki called it *Ko-och-e*. To the Little Lake and the Yokias it was *Ki-yi*. Manzanita is Spanish for "Little Apple."

Where to find it: Manzanitas of one species or another are found flourishing in a wide variety of habitats—in moist coastal regions, on rocky brushy ridges, in foothills and chaparral country, in the woods and in the mountains—in many California locations.

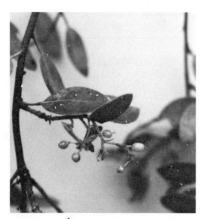

Manzanita

Sometimes, as on the picturesque Huckleberry Hill north of Monterey, where it's found in the shadows of the Monterey Pines, this common shrub grows in understory vegetation. Sometimes it's found fraternizing with Squaw Bush and Poison Oak or with Buckwheat, Mormon Tea, and Desert Peach.

How to know it when you see it: When it comes to describing this plant and its fruit, an account penned by the roving journalist Edwin Bryant way back in the 1840s doesn't fall far short. "We have met occasionally with a reddish berry called by the Californians, manzanita (little apple)," he wrote. "The berry is produced by small trees which stand in clumps, about ten or twelve feet in height, shedding their bark annually, leaving a smooth red surface. The flavor of the fruit is an agreeable acid, something like that of our apple."

Of course, Bryant might have gone on to note that these "clumps" of which he wrote sometimes grew so thick as to be impenetrable to either man or beast. He might have explained that other species of the same plant are much more tree-like in character. He could have mentioned how the bark of either type peeled off in thin curls, rather like the shavings that lie about a woodshop floor. He could have described the smooth polished wood as "burgundy-colored," rather than simply "red." He could have described the leaves of the plant as oval and pointed; its branches, twisted and tortured; its flowers as shaped like little urns; and its fruit as mealy. Still, today, as yesterday, his description, just as he penned it, is good enough to point the way to a stand of handsome Manzanitas, bedecked in berries waiting to be picked.

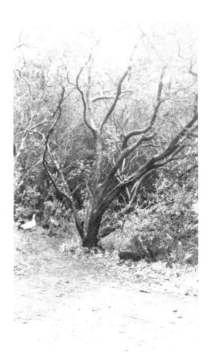

Manzanita

Its lore. To the California Indians, the Manzanita shrub was a marvelously multi-purpose plant. Among the many tribes who relished its nutritious berries and eagerly awaited their ripening year by year were the Calpellas, the Cahuillas, the Little Lakes, the Numlakis, the Wailakis, and the Keltas.

The Cahuillas, to whom the berries were a primary food source, sometimes made them into cider, as did the Yukis, the Shastas, the Wintun, and Yokuts, while the Numlakis dried them and ground them into a powder, which they cooked in hot ashes and served up like mush. Others ate them in cakes or stirred up in a mass with dry powdered salmon.

It was a joyous period for many Indians when the Manazanita berries ripened, a season of camaraderie and cheer. For some native Californians like the Concows, it was a celebration and a time of thanks-giving, a kind of holy day, marked by a feast they called the "big eat," at which they chanted and danced and consumed great quantities of fruit. To others, it was a time to go hunting for bears, for those great lumbering beasts were as fond of Manzanita fruit as the Indians, and were easy prey once they started munching berries. Still others, like the Viards, had a big feast in autumn, long after the berry-picking or bear-hunting days were over—a time for counting the blessings of spring and autumn, which included, of course, all the scarlet Manzanita-berries stashed away in wigwam attics.

Whether dined on by bears or bear hunters, the supply of the Manzanita fruit seemed so nearly never-ending that non-native observers couldn't help but note the economic aspects of such a wealth of food. According to his commentary, the amateur ethnographer, Stephen Powers, had seen Manzanita thickets in the Trinity Valley "wherein an acre could be selected that would yield more nutriment to human life, if the berries were all plucked, than the best acre of wheat ever grown in California, after the expenses of cultivation."

Like the berries, the wood of the Manazanita was highly valued. The Pomo used it to make a contrivance with which they could truck supplies that weighed as much as 200 pounds. It served as firewood to the Cahuilla. Others used it as a material from which to fashion tobacco pipes or tools and other wooden objects.

But it was the leaves of the Manzanita that the Indians seemed to consider most medicinal. From these the Little Lakes decocted a yellowish-red extract with which they dabbed themselves to ease away headaches. Some tribes mixed a good leaf lotion to treat the itch and inflammation of Poison Oak, while others mashed that same greenery to make poultices, reputedly soothing to various kinds of sores.

Today, even as some wild-food enthusiasts are trying out recipes for Manzanita cider, and survivalists are weighing the berry's value as a food, some modern herbalists are touting a Manzanita tincture or tea as a treatment for minor urinary complaints, kidney inflammations, water retention, and menstrual cramps, and an old-fashioned green-leaf poultice for an assortment of aches.

Comment: Years ago, two medical doctors, Dr. J. W. Hudson and Dr. B. C. Bellamy, who had treated the Indians of Round Valley at various times, reported several cases in which death followed over-consumption of Manzanita berries. Apparently the bowels of the victims had become blocked with great masses of fruit pulp and seed.

Large doses of Manzanita tea have been known to cause intestinal irritation.

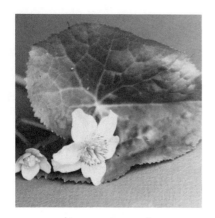

Marsh Marigold

MARSH MARIGOLD

Caltha palustris

Other names for the Marsh Marigold: Other names for this plant are Elkslip, American Cowslip, Kingcup, Blob, and Horse Blobs. One Spanish name for the Marigold is *Flameniquillo.*

Where to find it: The Marsh Marigold just barely qualifies as a wild-growing medicinal plant in California. It's found naturalized in a marsh near Forestville in lush Sonoma County. Another species of *Caltha*, which grows wild in some western states but *not* in California, is the very similar *Cleptosephalus*, whose medicinal uses are much the same.

How to know it when you see it: The most distinguishing feature of the highly medicinal little Marsh Marigold, which rarely grows taller than two feet, is its conspicuous, very bright green leaves, which lie somewhere between round and kidney-shaped, and are distinctly toothed at their margins. The flowers are showy too, white-petaled (its "petals" are really sepals), traced with blue on their undersides, yellow in their centers.

Its lore. Despite its visual charms and its reputation as a remedy, the lovely Marsh Marigold can be a very dangerous herb. Beware of its leaves. Although they're an excellent potherb *when cooked*, as tasty to many a wild-food enthusiast as the pickle-worthy Marsh Marigold flowers, it's not safe at all to eat them raw. And when applied to the skin, as they often are in a poultice for assorted rheumatoid pains, they can cause the flesh to blister and burn. Nonetheless, some modern herb buffs still believe that a small quantity of raw or dried leaf, especially combined with other herbs like Yerba Santa or Grindelia, is a good treatment for bronchial and sinus problems, and that the same warm-leaf poultice that's reputedly good for rheumatism is an acceptable treatment too for back pain and facial paralysis.

Comment: *Caltha palustris* is known to contain a highly irritating oil called anemonin.

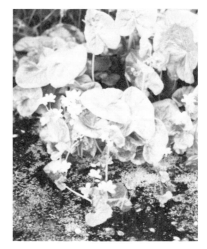

Marsh Marigold

MARSH WOUNDWORT

Stachys palustris

Other names for the Marsh Woundwort: Other names for this medicinal plant are Hedge-Nettle and Nettle Woundwort.

Where to find it: As its name implies, Marsh Woundwort is a true moisture lover. Look for it in damp meadows, by the sides of streams, in ditches, or at the edges of springs where it sometimes keeps company with ferns and Monkeyflowers.

How to know it when you see it: If you've even the slightest acquaintanceship with the mint family, of which the Woundworts are members, the square stems and the toothed leaves of this herb are instantly familiar. The natural inclination is to smell them at once, but any stranger to the so-called "hedge nettles" who follows that urge is in for a shock, for this is an herb with an odor that's not pleasantly minty but distinctly rank. It's rather a pretty plant despite its nettle-like hairs, and bears tiny rose-colored flowers that are veined with a darker red. These little blooms, with their lobed lower lips, have an interesting shape. Viewed straight on, as in silhouette, each one is like a cutout of Little Red Riding Hood with the hood of her cape pulled up over her head, her cloaked arms outspread in a gesture of wonder—rather like that evoked in the minds of children whose fancies conjure up such a vision.

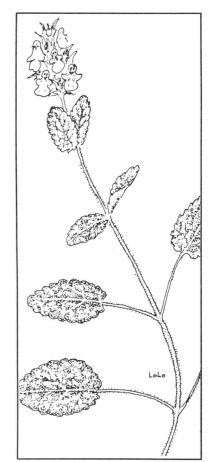

Marsh Woundwort

Its lore. California history is surprisingly silent on the subject of this old medicinal herb, one of several plants popularly known as "Woundworts." Yet here it grows; here the Indians must have seen it, must have touched and sampled it, must have found that its tubers were edible and that an infusion of its fresh leaves was a comfort to sore eyes. And surely the settlers recognized this herb as one from which their forebears had made poultices to apply to wounds to stop their bleeding and help them heal. Surely . . . and yet the early California records have little to say about *Stachys palustris*. In fact, there's more written about this plant today, now that foraging is fashionable, than there was for many decades.

Comment: No scientific evidence has been unearthed to support the early medicinal uses of *Stachys palustris*.

MEADOW RUE

Thalictrum polycarpum

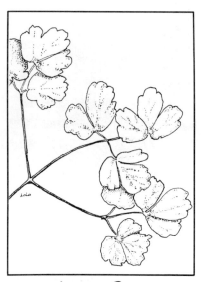

Meadow Rue

Other names for Meadow Rue: The Wailaki Indian name for the Meadow Rue was *Chin-dun-ga-chit*. The Little Lake called it *Ewe-shi-sha*, while to the Yuki it was *Hol-ga-shen*. Its Yokia name was *E-we buch-o-a*.

Where to find it: Most species of Meadow Rue, including also the so-called Few-flowered and Fendler's, are moisture lovers, fond of thickets and streams and other damp spots.

How to know it when you see it: Don't just see it; smell it. If it's aromatic, if you find yourself leaning over to catch its scent a second time, it may well be Meadow Rue. The plant is generally about three or four feet in height, bears finely divided leaves, and inconspicuous flowers.

Its lore. Much of the interesting lore of this old Indian herb is hinted at by its name. When translated, its Yuki moniker, *Hol-ga-shen*, and that of the Yokia, *E-we buch-o-a*, both mean "Coyote Angelica." By the California Indians, for whom true Angelica was doubtless the most respected medicinal herb of all the plants they knew, the coyote was considered the most cunning of all creatures. Since this was true, it follows that a plant had to be considered very special in order to earn the label "Coyote Angelica." The meadow rue qualified; it was so special that its virtues, like those of its namesakes, smacked of the world of magic and the realm of spirit. It was almost as aromatic as Angelica; that in itself was like an omen. And yet, unlike Angelica, which was a gentle talisman, it was dangerously poisonous. Wasn't this a known fact? Hadn't a little white child once died from mistaking the stem of one for the stem of the other?

But wasn't it also true that the coyote was so cunning he could consume that poisonous plant and not be fazed by his folly? Couldn't he lope away unscathed after he'd gnawed at its lethal stems? And wasn't there a sense in which the immunity of the coyote only served to render the plant all the more dangerous to anyone else—like those who were already dead and buried, whose hard-won rest would be interrupted by terrible nightmares if the Coyote Angelica plant was allowed to grow on their graves? Didn't the living Wailakis know this full well and thereby act upon their knowledge? Wasn't it true that when the deceased would suddenly and inexplicably cross their minds they would hasten to the burial ground and uproot the Meadow Rue, which, according to their calculations, they were almost sure to find growing over the graves? They'd dig it up at once and wash their heads in the juice from the crushed stems and crumbled leaves, as a kind of propitiation rite, to make certain that the deceased could rest well once more.

But the juice of the Meadow Rue was more than a cure for the bad dreams of the dead. Oddly enough, the same application that could quell those native nightmares could soothe the common headaches of the living, just as surely as if it were some beneficent decoction from an ordinary herb, wholly unadulterated by the coyote's cunning.

MESQUITE

Prosopis juliflora

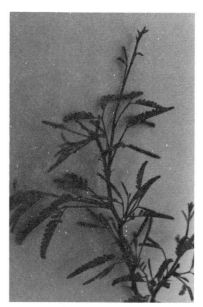

Mesquite

Other names for the Mesquite Tree: Other English names for this hardy tree are Honey Mesquite and Western Honey Mesquite. The Cahuilla name for the Mesquite was *Ily*.

Where to find it: As true a westerner as any character in a Zane Grey novel, at home especially in the Colorado and Mojave Deserts, the familiar old Mesquite tree thrives in Creosote Bush Scrub, on the dry edges of alkali sinks, in desert washes, and in other low places below 3,000 feet.

How to know it when you see it: Sometimes a large shrub, sometimes a small tree, reaching heights between twenty and fifty feet, the Mesquite is a common plant of arid places. Its leaves, which are deciduous, are divided into many small leaflets. Its small, fragrant flowers, borne in slender spikes like bottle brushes for very long vessels, are variously described as "greenish-yellow," and "greenish-white." Its fruits, which are about six inches long, are flat and pod-like; its branches are arched; and its thirsty roots are incredibly long, sometimes reaching sixty feet into the ground.

Its lore. From the looks of it, there's nothing so special about this tree, nothing to endear it to any poet or romancer who eyes the moon through a veil of thorny Mesquite branches. It's not a plant of grand proportions; it's not especially beautiful. The shade it casts, welcome as it is in arid places, is minimal compared to that of other California trees. Yet none other afforded the long, sweet pods, from which the desert tribes ground the flour that filled their bellies and nourished their bodies. None other inspired the shamans to such supernatural heights as they prayed for blessed crops and brimming larders, for the bounty of the tribal groves. No other tree gave rise to religious devotions like those which took place at the *kish'amna'a*, the ceremonial house, where all members of a certain lineage had to eat and pray together before they went to gather the new year's harvest. None other served as ingredients for the wonderful little Mesquite cakes the Cahuilla gave to the Dieguenos or the Luisenos when they attended their fiestas. (No other gift was quite so fitting, no other cake so sweet.) Nor did any other tree or shrub ever drive the desert tribes to indulge in private ownership as did this commonplace shrub. *This is the grove of my family; here we will harvest our own pods. That is the grove of yours. Let us not exceed our boundaries. Let us take only that which is ours.*

But the Mesquite was more than a primary source of food for the Indians of the California desert. It was a source too of a fiber from which to make infant diapers and other useful items. It was a provider of building material: wood for making bows, corner posts for houses, and rafters from which to hang an assortment of supplies. It was fuel, and as such, it was burned to bake pottery, to keep bodies warm, to cook meals, and to ready the sweathouse for gatherings of the people. Furthermore, it was a virtual treasury of medicines. Sometimes it was a treatment to rid the head of vermin, in which case the clear gum that exuded from cuts in the shrub's smooth trunk was first mixed with mud, then applied to the head as a wonder-working pack. Sometimes it was a soothing fresh-leaf lotion for irritated eyes. Sometimes it was a poultice, or a plaster, or a salve. Always it was a blessing and a boon—the little tree that made life tenable for the desert tribes of yesterday.

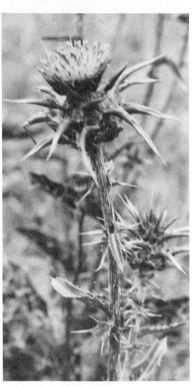

Milk Thistle

MILK THISTLE

Silybum marianum

Other names for the Milk Thistle: This old medicinal plant is also known as Marian Thistle and Mothers' Milk Plant.

Where to find it: A native of the Mediterranean region, Milk Thistle is a common weed in pastures and waste places in many California locations.

How to know it when you see it: As tall and erect as a foot soldier, prickled and crinkly from top to bottom, there's no plant more easily identified than this formidable-looking old stand-by among medicinal herbs. Even its purplish flowers, reminiscent of fine silk tassels themselves, are surrounded by spines. But its stickery, heavily-lobed leaves are traced with veins of the purest milky white, and this is clear testimony, according to the ancient Doctrine of Signatures, that here's a medicament meant for the gentle job of increasing lactation in nursing mothers. It's as simple as that.

Its lore. Despite the clear "signature" it bore (which might as well have been written in mothers' milk, as far as some early herbalists were concerned) and despite the fact that its praise had been sung since the days of the Roman naturalist, Pliny, Milk Thistle was apparently never a really popular medicinal herb in early California. Still, this is a plant with a long tradition of medicinal use, and one that's ironically looked upon more kindly by today's herbalists, survivalists, and wild-food enthusiasts than it was by the the early settlers of the nineteenth century. Its age-old uses are well worth recounting.

There was a time when wet nurses in Europe religiously included this herb in the special diets they employed to ensure their supply of milk. In fact, the term "religiously," used here, is a true double entendre. It was a common belief in those days that the reason the herb increased lactation—the reason that the prickly leaves were traced with those telltale white veins to begin with—was that drops of milk from the Virgin Mary's breasts had fallen upon them as she'd nursed the holy infant, Jesus. Almost equally popular was another Marian legend, according to which the vein-tracing milk fell from her breasts, not while she was nursing, but as she was cutting a bit of the thistle itself to feed it as fodder to the little donkey who bore her and her babe on down the road.

As to the aforementioned Pliny, who penned his herbal reflections way back in the first-century A.D., that gentleman boldly averred that this well-armored plant was "excellent for carrying off bile," an opinion that's actually been corroborated by current research. The truth is that the fruit of the Milk Thistle contains a chemical substance called silymarin, which does indeed have a restorative effect upon the liver. It stimulates the growth of new cells, thereby promoting healthy self-repair. For this reason, the herb, which never played an important role in early California folk medicine, is now recognized as one of the most beneficent medicinal plants known to humankind. It supplies an antidote to the "death cap" mushroom, which kills by destroying the liver cells of those who've ingested it; and it yields a regenerative drug which is useful in treating hepatitis and cirrhosis of the liver.

Enthralled by these discoveries, modern herbalists are reconsidering some of the other traditional uses of this old herb. These are many, for at one time or another, Milk Thistle has been employed to treat infertility, to ease flatulence, to cure an acid stomach, to aid in digestion, to soothe gastritis, and to treat diarrhea and dysentery. Besides all this, despite its thorns (which, of course need to be removed before it's served up for dinner), Milk Thistle is also quite edible, a tasty salad green or cooked vegetable, good for the appetite, good for digestion.

MILKWEED

Asclepias speciosa

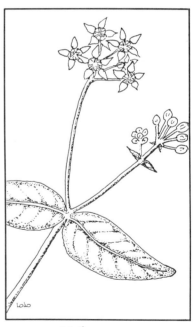

Milkweed

Other names for Milkweed: Other English names are Common Milkweed and Showy Milkweed. The Cahuilla called it *Kivat* or *Kyal*. To the Yuki it was *Ch'a-ak*, to the Concow, *Bo-ko*, and to the Little Lake it was *G-to-la*. The Spanish name for the plant is *Lechones*.

Where to find it: *Asclepias speciosa* favors valleys and streamside locations at altitudes that range from sea level to 6,000 feet.

How to know it when you see it: The leaves of *A. speciosa*, which are arranged in opposite pairs, are whitish, velvety to the touch, and oval to oblong in shape. The stem is simple and erect. The unique flowers of pinkish-white or pearly pink, have projecting "hoods" and are clustered in great round balls, a showy sight. The plant generally ranges in height from one to four feet, which means it's much the same size as its relative, *A. eriocarpa*, another popular medicinal Milkweed found in California. (See Indian Milkweed.)

Its lore. What was true of other medicinal Milkweeds was true of this one too. Its sticky juice served as an ingredient in a salve for sores, cuts, warts, and ringworm; its seeds were included in a recipe for rattlesnake bites; its roots went to make a good measle tea and a poultice for sprained ankles. Yet, for whatever reasons, *Asclepias speciosa* appears to have some purposes that kindred herbs haven't always shared, purposes that time has not obliterated. After centuries of such use by Indians and settlers alike, this much-respected Milkweed is still employed as a remedy for urinary problems and kidney weaknesses. It's reputed to stimulate perspiration, to soften excess mucus, and to stimulate free expectoration. Herbalists warmly tout it still, just as they did when America was young.

Comment: Like other native Milkweed plants, *A. speciosa* is toxic to livestock.

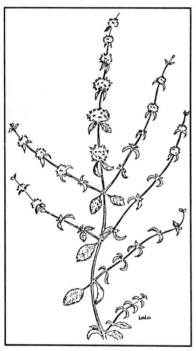

Pennyroyal

MINT

Mentha spp.

Other names for Mint: *M. arvensis* is known variously as Poleo Mint, Brook Mint, Indian Mint, Corn Mint, Horse Mint, Field Mint, and Wild Mint. *M. piperita* is best known as Peppermint, *M. pulegium* as Pennyroyal, and *M. spicata* as Spearmint. The Spanish name for Mint is *Menta*.

Where to find it: All of these mints thrive in damp meadows, along the sides of streams and ditches, and around the margins of springs where they sometimes keep company with other moisture-loving plants like the beautiful Scarlet Monkeyflower. Poleo mint, the only one of these herbs thought to be native to the American West and the one most apt to tolerate the higher altitudes, is common in many California locations. Peppermint, a mint of the lower altitudes, is naturalized only occasionally. Pennyroyal is a familiar herb in many California counties including San Diego, Monterey, Santa Clara, Sonoma, Mendocino, Marin, and Humboldt. Spearmint grows in moist fields and meadows in various parts of the state.

How to know it when you see it: All of these herbs are perennials; all boast the square stems so typical of mints; all spread by means of runners. Spearmint reaches heights up to four feet, all the others up to three. The flowers of Peppermint are usually purplish-rose; those of Spearmint, which grow in whorls and form a spike, are generally lavender. Poleo Mint and Pennyroyal are the least coarse-looking of these four mints. Neither of them flower in terminal spikes as do many of their kin, but rather in the axils of their upper leaves, which are smoother and less crinkly than Spearmint's, almost fragile-looking in comparison.

Its lore. The mint that was prized by the the early Spanish settlers, grown especially in the gardens of that prominent Californio, Jose M. de Estudillo, who traded in herbs as some men did in hides or gold, was most probably Peppermint or Spearmint. Even today these two are the best known species of *mentha*, popular herbs of the dooryard, commercially important, aromatic, medicinal, and good tasting. But European Pennyroyal has also been a much-favored herb in California for many years. Believed to have been cultivated here first by the mission padres, it brought its good reputation with it when it came from the old-country where it was once thought capable of curing headaches, relieving stomach-aches, improving eyesight, erasing the marks of bruises and black eyes, cleansing ulcers and burns, and making life easier for lepers.

All these mints are still among the favorite herbs used by modern herbalists and folk medicine buffs. Peppermint, a common ingredient in many commercial candies, medicines, liqueurs, and cigarettes, still serves as an old stand-by home remedy to aid digestion, relieve heartburn, and ward off seasickness. The less potent Spearmint more often serves as a culinary herb, especially to enhance lamb dishes. Pennyroyal, which, because of its strong volatile oil can be dangerous, is still sometimes used to promote menstruation, to ease fevers, and to treat stomach and bowel upsets. Poleo, our native western mint, can be made into a delicious tea, a wonderful after-dinner drink that's relaxing, tonic, and good for the digestion.

Warning: Pennyroyal, *Mentha pulegium*, can be a dangerous herb if used in excess. It contains the toxin pulegone, a volatile oil that is harmful when consumed in large amounts. Symptoms of injudicious use (which can result in liver damage) are vomiting, delirium, respiratory difficulty, and unconsciousness. The commercial product called Pennyroyal Oil is not meant for human consumption.

MISTLETOE

Phoradendron spp. and *Viscum album*

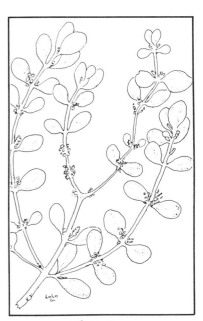

Mistletoe

Other names for Mistletoe: *Phoradendron* species are called American Mistletoe. *Viscum album* is called European Mistletoe. Both plants are popularly known as Golden Bough. The Little Lake Indians called Mistletoe *Tsi ma-ar-she*. To the Cahuilla it was *Chayal*.

Where to find it: A scrubby and clumpy parasitic plant, often highly destructive to the trees that are its reluctant hosts, American Mistletoe is a common sight in orchards and woodlands in many parts of California, where it clings uninvited to the branches of Oaks and Junipers and many deciduous trees, sometimes embedded deeply in the crooks of their limbs.

European Mistletoe, *Viscum album*, unknown in California before the coming of the white man, is naturalized only in Sonoma County, where it was introduced at the beginning of the twentieth century and is still found growing in some of the county's few remaining apple orchards.

How to know it when you see it: When viewed from a distance, a Mistletoe plant looks like a clump of greenery that has been tied together and tossed at random up into the branches of the gnarled Oaks where it so often dwells. At close range the plant is markedly artificial-looking. The thick opposite leaves of the most typical specimens might as well be cutouts from scraps of thick shoe leather. (Shoe leather that's been dyed green and turned wrong-side-up so that it's as soft to the touch as that popular fabric called suede cloth.) Before they ripen, at which time they turn white, the small single-seeded berries of the plant are the self-same rich moss-green as are its leaves and the stems, and this single-color sameness renders it all the more artificial-looking. Parasite that it is, and a poisonous one at that, it's an attractive plant, and, in light of the legends that surround it, a fitting decoration at Christmastime.

Its lore. Some of the California Indians, the Wintun, for example, smoked Oak Mistletoe in lieu of tobacco. Others used the plant as an effective toothache remedy, deemed all the more powerful if they'd found it growing on a Buckeye tree, a placement that was thought to lend it special efficacy. It was also considered an effective herb at the time of childbirth and a good remedy for tardy menstruation.

Settlers may have tried these treatments too. In fact, since *Phoradendron* is common in other parts of the country as well, and was, therefore, familiar to them already, they may even have been using the plant medicinally before they made the trek westward. In the nineteenth century many Americans were still reared on old-country folklore and schooled in old-country herbology, and hence were inclined to look with interest upon this species that shared so many characteristics with the legendary European Mistletoe. Woven into the themes of countless old fairy tales and bedtime stories, the old-world species, *Viscum album*, which the Romans and the Celts had looked upon as a supernatural sign of fertility, had also been considered a matchless medicament, useful in treating every sort of ailment from barrenness to tuberculosis, from palsy to poisoning, from strokes to epilepsy, from unrequited-love sickness to plain old insomnia. It was not surprising that some of the lore of the old-world Mistletoe attached itself to its American counterpart and clung there for many years as tenaciously as the plant itself clings to the Oaks that serve as its unwilling hosts.

Even today, while most herbalists avoid its use as a medicinal plant, Mistletoe still plays a role in the folklore of America, just as it does in old-world lands. Come Christmastime, its greenery still graces ceilings and doorways, where it's tacked amidst Angel's hair and tinsel, bells and blown glass. Romantic lovers still stand beneath it and seal their intentions with a kiss.

Comment: Although there is reportedly some evidence that certain old claims made for American Mistletoe may have had basis in fact—that the plant may possess properties that could induce menstruation, relax nervous tension, and increase blood pressure—most herbalists warn that this herb is not to be taken internally. All parts of this plant are toxic. Symptoms of Mistletoe poisoning include stomach cramps, intestinal pains, diarrhea, slowing pulse, vomiting, delirium, abortion, hallucination, and heart failure. When used as Christmas decorations, the plant should be kept well out of the reach of children and animals.

MORMON TEA

Ephedra

Other names for Mormon Tea: Other English names for Mormon Tea are Mexican Tea, Squaw Tea, Brigham Tea, Teamsters Tea, Desert Tea, Joint Fir, Miner's Tea, Cowboy Tea, American Ephedra, and Whorehouse Tea. The Cahuilla called this plant *Tutut*. To California's hispanic population it's popularly known as both *Canutillo* and *Popotillo*.

Where to find it: Always at home with Pinyon, Rabbitbrush, and Creosote Bush, sometimes found in the company of Joshua Trees, Buffaloberry, Bitterbrush, and Cholla, or amongst the Wild Currants, the Buckwheat, and Manzanita, this homely plant is widely distributed throughout the arid sections of the state. Where the land is forbidding, there it grows; there it thrives; there it serves the human beings who share its habitat, just as it has for centuries on end.

How to know it when you see it: Although many a southwesterner's voice might rise to sing the praises of its fine refreshing tea, few would describe this plant as a lovely one. Growing sometimes to a height of four feet, sometimes erect, sometimes creeping, it's nonetheless a stunted-looking shrub, weather-beaten, unkempt, so profusely-branched it's rather like a broom. Its skinny, barkless stems of dull greenish-blue are jointed; its leaves, growing in opposite pairs or in whorls of three, are scaly; its nondescript flowers are yellowish-green.

Its lore. Homely though it is, "leggy as a spider," according to one old man who uses it still, Mormon Tea could rightly be called "an herb for all people." As the makings of a good drink, a fine stem tea, or a tasty food, ground meal for mush, or as a remedy for a list of ailments that ranged from stomach-aches to the "French disease" (syphilis), this plant was used not only by desert Indians but by the Spanish settlers who were their neighbors. So too by adventurers, soldiers, miners, teamsters, cowboys, and by all those ordinary settlers who made the trip cross-country, thirsty for a good substitute for store-bought tea and in dire need of medicine for the motley ills that troubled them.

In the nineteenth century, when it reached its peak of popularity, the famous tea of this scraggly old wilding was administered regularly for kidney problems, bladder complaints, cramps, headaches, fevers, common colds, arthritis, and rheumatism, while poultices and ointments of dried and pulverized twigs were applied religiously to burns and sores, ulcers and swellings, animal bites, and rashes of every variety.

Even today many southern Californians are staunch in their insistence that there's no more health-giving potion on the face of Mother Earth than a brimming cup of good old-fashioned, fresh-brewed Mormon Tea, made from a plant for which they've gone out foraging themselves. It's as if the personal touch, the seeking, the picking, and all the preparation add something special to its refreshing taste and its tonic effects.

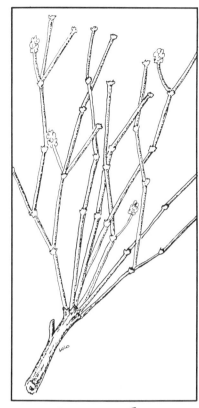

Mormon-Tea

MULE EARS

Wyethia longicaulis

Other names for Mule Ears: This plant is often referred to as simply "Sunflower." The Yuki Indians used to call it *Bish-non.* To the Wailaki it was *Cha-la,* to the Little Lake, *Chi-lam,* while to the Yokia it was *De-wish-a-lum.*

Where to find it: This common member of the Sunflower family is at home in open woods, on exposed ridges, on the coastal prairies, and in mixed evergreen forests in several northern California counties. It favors altitudes that range from 2,500 to 5,000 feet.

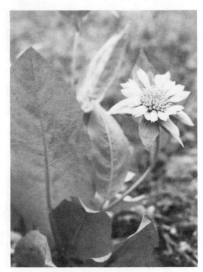

Mule Ears

How to know it when you see it: This perennial herb, two feet tall, bears rather slender stems, bright yellow ray flowers that are generally two to four inches in diameter, and broad lanceolate leaves reminiscent of the ears of mules, each of which measure from twelve to eighteen inches long.

Its lore. Every part of this sunny plant, but most especially its richly aromatic root, is pervaded with a warming balsamic oil, that was once much-prized for its medicinal properties. When they were racked by rheumatic pains, or they'd been burned, or they were vexed by running sores, the Yuki Indians, the Little Lake, the Yokia, and the Wailaki all turned to this herb for comfort. Sometimes, especially for their aches, they baked its medicinal root in hot ashes and applied it in the form of a poultice. At other times they dried it and ground it to a powder, which they moistened and applied as a kind of salve. Or they made a fine root decoction and used it as a wash for headaches and sore eyes. As the source of a poultice, a powder, or a wash, and sometimes even as a source of food, the northern tribes prized this yellow-flowered plant of many names.

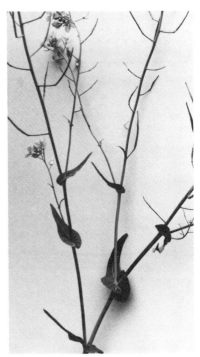

Field Mustard

MUSTARD

Brassica nigra and *Sisymbrium officinale*

Other names for Mustard: *Brassica nigra* is best known as Black Mustard. *Sisymbrium officinale* is popularly called Hedge Mustard, Scrambling Rocket, and Singer's Plant.

Where to find it: Natives of Europe, both of these species thrive now in various waste places all over the United States and throughout the state of California: in fields, on roadsides, and on grassy slopes.

Mustard used to grow so profusely around the Mission Santa Clara that, according to Edwin Bryant, who visited there in the 1840s, "it is with difficulty that a horse can penetrate through it."

How to know it when you see it: Hedge Mustard is an annual or biennial plant with many slender stems, deeply dissected leaves, and flowers that grow in racemes. Black Mustard, which reaches a height of six feet, bears leaves that are considerably smaller and narrower at the top of the plant than at the bottom. The flowers of both plants are yellow and are typically four-petaled.

Its lore. Black Mustard (called "black" because of its small dark seeds) is the plant that afforded the settlers one of the most famous "treatments" in the annals of American folk medicine, the much-extolled, often effective, sometimes skin-blistering Mustard plaster with which they treated colds, coughs, bronchitis, and pluerisy. This pasty medicament, a concoction of flour, water, and powdered mustard, was spread between two pieces of fabric, usually flannel, and applied externally to the chest of the "victim." Sometimes it was a home remedy, self-prescribed or administered by some artless "kitchen shaman," but just as often it was concocted on a doctor's orders.

According to one native daughter, Natlee Kenoyer, the Mustard plaster was still in common usage in California hospitals as late as 1920, when it was finally replaced by more modern treatments for chest congestion. A writer and a teacher of horsemanship nowadays (still riding at the age of 82!), for many years she was a registered nurse in a Fresno hospital, and well remembers how frequently the staff used to turn to this old stand-by remedy. "We mixed one part Mustard with four parts flour," she explains. "We folded it up like an envelope, applied it every three to four hours, and left it on from three to five minutes at a time. Afterward we rubbed the chest with camphorated oil. Maybe it was just psychological but it sure did seem to work."

Though scarcely a popular remedy now, an external application of *Brassica nigra* is not entirely a thing of the past. Some modern advocates of old-fashioned herbal remedies like Dennis Moneymaker of Sonoma County, who turned to a Mustard plaster to ease the lingering symptoms of a case of pneumonia, are convinced that this age-old treatment is more than a placebo.

Perhaps not so popular a household remedy as Black Mustard was (and still is with people like Dennis), it was Hedge Mustard that once commanded the respect of singers, poets, and speakers, to whom a bout with laryngitis was an unspeakable bane. Its popularity had probably peaked in the eighteenth century, long before settlers came roving into California from the eastern states, but even at that later date most people still believed that there was no remedy more likely to initiate a speedy return of the lost voice. This herb was also used to treat colds, pleurisy, sciatica, canker sores, and other common ills.

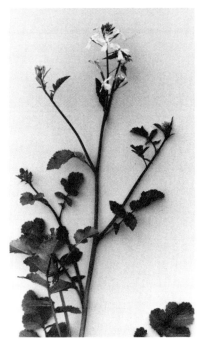

Shortpod Mustard

Comment: In light of the fact that Mustard greens are a well-known food, and Mustard seed is the source of one of our most popular and widely-used condiments, it goes without saying that, when judiciously used, Mustard is not a dangerous herb. However, like many other foods, it can be harmful under certain circumstances. If an excess of raw Mustard is consumed it can cause extreme irritation of the intestinal tract and symptoms that include vomiting and diarrhea. Furthermore, Mustard plasters can burn and blister the skin, and pure Mustard oil can severely injure the human eye.

NETTLE

Urtica spp.

Other names for Nettle: Another popular English name for this herb is Stinging Nettle. Its Spanish name is *Ortiga*. To the Cahuilla it was *Chikishlyam*.

Where to find it: Nettles appear to be happiest in cool, moist, and shady locations. *Urtica holosericea*, the species known to the desert Indians, is found in low damp places at altitudes below 9,000 feet. Sometimes, however, as evidenced by its use there, it thrives on the desert's edge. *U. serra* is found in wet places at altitudes between 5,000 and 10,000 feet. Both *U. lyallii* and *U. californica* favor coastal locations, while the Dwarf Nettle, *U. urens*, a naturalized European found growing as a weed, most often appears uninvited in gardens and orchards.

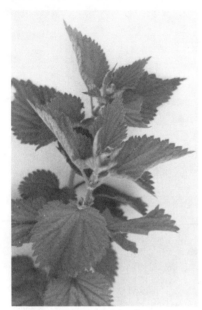

Stinging Nettle

How to know it when you see it: The small, light green flowers of the Stinging Nettle, perhaps its most distinguishing features, are borne in decorative loosely-hanging spikes that furl out in all directions like strings of beads on a swinging chandelier. The opposite leaves of the plant, which are velvety-looking, heart-shaped, rough-surfaced, and coarsely-toothed, are covered with stinging bristles, as are its stems. Stinging Nettles vary in size according to species, some reaching a height of seven feet.

Its lore. The Cahuilla Indians once used this plant as a cure for rheumatism and stiff muscles, a cure that was, notably, not without its wages. Afflicted feet were treated by applying nettles directly to the flesh and then swathing both feet and the sorely stinging mass in cloth. The treatment for headaches and rheumatic pains was much the same, an operation so painful one can't help wondering if the remedy wasn't a great deal worse than the ailments cured.

This herb is still in good repute today. A strong leaf infusion is touted by some modern herbalists as a hair tonic that stimulates growth and cures dandruff; a tea of the foliage is believed to ease the symptoms of colds, bronchitis, and excessive menstruation; a fresh-leaf poultice is said to be a pain reliever.

Warning: Never collect Nettle leaves without having first armored yourself with a good thick pair of gloves. The plant's stingers can cause extreme discomfort. Symptoms of skin penetration are reddening, itching, burning, and swelling. Contact with the herb, which can also trigger a bout of hay fever, has been known to cause tremors and convulsions in hunting dogs.

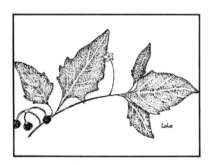

Nightshade

NIGHTSHADE

Solanum spp.

Other names for Nightshade: The Numlaki name for the Nightshade was *Mon-uk*. To the Cahuilla it was *Ayka'kal.*

Where to find it: The Nightshade that was used medicinally by the Cahuilla, *Solanum douglasi,* is found from Monterey County to coastal southern California. Dwelling even in the arid deserts, it favors canyons and partly shaded slopes at altitudes below 5,000 feet. The Numlaki's *Mon-uk* (*S. nigrum*), however, occurs often as a garden weed in northern California.

How to know it when you see it: This is a low, spreading plant, which measures from one to two or three feet across, bears ovate to elliptic-ovate leaves that are irregularly toothed, tiny whitish flowers, and conspicuous bluish-black berries.

Its lore. The Nightshade's official name, *Solanum,* comes from the Latin, *solamen,* which means "quieting," a clue that this genus has long been known to possess narcotic properties. To the desert Indians, who shared its habitat, however, it was not used as a tranquilizer as might be supposed, but as a trusted eye medicament. The juice of the little dark berry, sometimes squeezed full-strength directly into the eye, sometimes first diluted, was administered as a treatment for cases of strain, pink eye, and poor vision.

OAKS

Quercus spp.

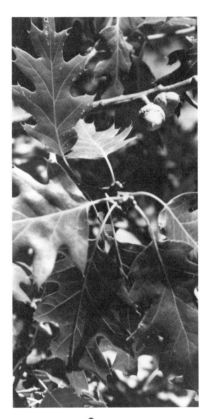

Oak

Other names for California's Oaks: Canyon Live Oak, Blue Oak, Scrub Oak (also called Curl-leaf Scrub Oak), Pacific Post Oak (also called Oregon Oak), California Black Oak, California White Oak, and Valley Oak (also called Valley White Oak). The Yuki name for the California Black Oak was *Nun*. The Little Lake called it *Du-she ka-la*. The Pomo name for the Scrub Oak was *Bat-son*, while the Cahuilla called it *Pawish*. The Yuki name for the Oregon Oak was *Ma-le*. The Spanish name for Oak is *Encino*.

Where to find them: Barring only certain desert and high mountain places, Oaks of one variety or another are found growing almost everywhere in the state.

The Canyon Live Oak, which abides on canyon floors, in narrow gullies and on terraces of rock, is the most widely distributed of these trees, ranging as it does all the way from Oregon down into Baja California. As its common name so clearly indicates, the Coast Live Oak, thriving from Sonoma County to Santa Barbara County, is practically restricted to the Coast Ranges. The Blue Oak is a foothill dweller found at altitudes below 4,000 feet.

How to know them when you see them: While the great, spreading California White Oak grows to a height of eighty feet, the Scrub Oak is often only three to eight feet tall. But not only is there a tremendous variation in the size of the Oak species that populate the state, there is a great difference in the size and shape of their leaves as well. As was noted by the awestruck naturalist Thomas Nuttall, who was the first of his ilk to visit California, some members of this genus weren't Oak-like at all, but instead had "leaves like a holly."

To certain early sojourners the California Oaks were known as much for their beauty as for their utility. The journalist, Edwin Bryant, never forgot those he saw here in the 1840s, in woods that he referred to poetically as "parks," as if they'd been purposefully planted and tended for the benefit of the yet-to-come public. "Proceeding with our journey," he wrote, "we traveled fifteen miles over a flat plain, timbered with groves and parks of evergreen oaks . . . Numerous birds flitted from tree to tree, making the groves musical with their harmonious notes. The black-tailed deer bounded frequently across our path, and the lurking and stealthy coyotes were continually in view."

But one can't necessarily name a tree by its ambience. In the light of all the variation between one Oak and another, the best way to identify a wilding as a species of *Quercus* is by the presence of the the telltale acorn, which, despite certain differences from species to species, is always recognizable for what it is.

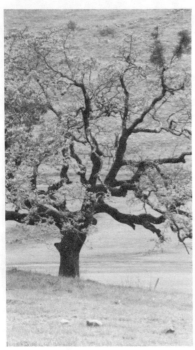

Oak

Its lore. It's odd that the Oak's role in California folk medicine is so often ignored, for to many of the early residents of the land the genus *Quercus* was a trusted remedy. The Yukis, for example, used the bark of the Valley Oak as a treatment for diarrhea, the Cahuillas made a fine antiseptic wash from the ashes of burnt Oak wood, and settlers concocted a healing salve from Oak bark and lard.

Perhaps these medicinal uses were left unmentioned simply because their value seemed insignificant when compared to the importance of the food the Oak yielded. With up to 5,000 pounds of acorns representing only one year's supply for a single Indian family, it's easy to see why its position as the source of a most vital staple was always its greatest claim to fame. Even to those desert tribes to whom the acorn mattered less than it did to the coastal Indians, this fruit of the Oak was still a vital food and a pivotal force in the community. Among the Cahuillas, for example, the shamans (the *puvalam*) conducted countless ceremonies meant to ensure the safety and productivity of the more or less privately-owned groves, each of which was called *Meki'i'wah*—a word meaning "the place that waits for me." And it's said that the failure of one year's acorn crop was so serious a matter to another tribe, the Luiseno, that it sometimes led to warfare.

But as was often the case with a food that was so critical to the Indians as to provoke territorialism and give rise to ritual, there was considerable overlapping of the medicinal, spiritual, and nutritional aspects of the acorn. A food without which one cannot survive becomes sacred to the survivors. Its impact is healthgiving and lifegiving, and therefore it is holy, in the strictest sense of these terms. In the eyes of the native Americans, that which is holy makes way for healing. Hence, to most tribes of California Indians, there was no food purer, no substance less tainted or more apt to promote wellbeing than the acorn, its meal, its gruel, or its mush.

To the sun-worshipping Costanoans (the coast people), as to the northern Shoshoneans, acorns were an acceptable offering at the ritual dances of the winter solstice. With other tribes, a thin acorn soup was the only food pure enough to be consumed by fasting shamans as they steeped themselves in prayer and readied themselves to heal the sick. It was the only substance fit to touch the lips of mothers giving birth, or young girls during the days that they were menstruating, or young boys at the time they were ushered into manhood. As the acorn was holy and healing, it was obviously a profoundly medicinal substance even when thought of largely as a food. As such it rates more attention in the annals of California folk medicine than it usually gets.

Some modern herbalists use an Oak bark tea as a gargle for scratchy throats or sore gums and a decoction of bark and twigs as a treatment for minor burns. Survivalists and backpackers miles from the nearest drugstore favor the plant as an ever-available antiseptic, good for treating all sorts of backwoods vexations. A strong bark decoction is used for cuts and scratches and campfire burns; mashed leaves make a good bolus to apply to insect bites; a bit of chewed bark is said to ease away a minor toothache.

Comments: All of California's sixteen species of native Oaks bear edible acorns. Before this favorite food of the California Indians is rendered edible, however, it must be carefully leached under running water so that the toxic tannin can be removed.

Cattle and sheep are occasionally poisoned by browsing on the young leaves and buds of various Oaks. Symptoms are poor appetite, thirst, swelling, urination, constipation, bloody stools, and kidney dysfunction that may ultimately lead to death. Since the bitterness of raw nuts precludes their overconsumption, acorns do not generally pose a danger to human beings.

OREGON ASH

Fraxinus latifolia

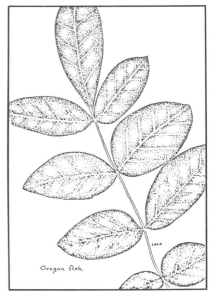

Oregon Ash

Other names for the Oregon Ash: The Yokian name for the Oregon Ash was *galam*, while the Yuki called it *Pok*.

Where to find it: Sometimes keeping company with Box Elder, Cottonwoods, Willows, and Black Walnut trees, this moisture lover dwells in canyons, in riverlands, or by the sides of streams at altitudes up to 5,500 feet.

How to know it when you see it: The leaves of the Oregon Ash are comprised of five to seven ovate leaflets, usually smooth-margined or only finely toothed, which measure from three to six inches long and from one to one and a half inches wide. The tree itself measures as much as seventy-five feet in height and three feet in diameter.

Its lore. A source of fuel to several tribes of Indians, a source too of fine wood from which to fashion such valuable items as canes and staffs, handles of tools, and pipes to smoke, the Oregon Ash also furnished a valuable medicament. The Yokias dug up a portion of the potent fresh roots, mashed them thoroughly and applied them poultice-fashion to snakebites and to flesh wounds made by the bears that were once so common in California.

Settlers also made medicinal use of the Oregon Ash. This was probably the tree to which early Sutter's Fort resident, Heinrich Lienhard, was referring when he mentioned a plant called "California Ash," a remedy that proved salvific to a certain ailing forty-niner who called on him for help. "Once when Thomen stopped on his way back from the mines," Lienhard wrote in his famous memoirs, " he was so sick that I made him a tea brewed from the roots of the California Ash. He believed it would cure him, and it did make him well."

OUR LORD'S CANDLE

Yucca whipplei

Other names for Our Lord's Candle: Other English names for this plant are Spanish Bayonet, Adam's-needle, Bear Grass, and Quixote Plant. The Cahuilla name for Our Lord's Candle was *Panu'ul*.

Where to find it: Not really the cactus that most tourists assume it to be, Our Lord's Candle does flourish in the same desert-like places where cactus plants

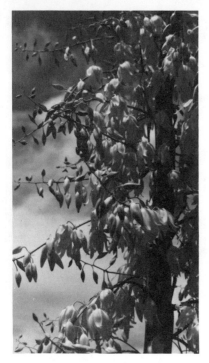

Our Lord's Candle

thrive. It's found growing on dry and rocky slopes at altitudes between 1,000 and 4,000 feet, in chaparral plant communities, in coastal sage and Creosote Bush scrub, especially in the southern section of the state.

How to know it when you see it: Often used as an ornamental plant, conspicuous only when it's flowering and fruiting (after which time its life is over), *Y. whipplei* has long, narrow leaves that are stiff and sharp, and cream-colored, lily-like flowers that appear on a thick, tall, upward-thrusting stalk.

Its lore. To the Diegueno Indians the Yucca plants afforded the fiber from which saddle blankets were manufactured. To other desert tribes, such as the Cahuilla, the stalks and flowers and fleshy fruits of Our Lord's Candle were a fine food, sometimes described as squash-like. To these and other Indians, the roots of these denizens of arid places served sometimes as an all-purpose sudsing agent, sometimes as a medicament for minor skin problems, and sometimes, unlikely though it may seem, as the chief ingredient in a tincture that was supposed to be good for gonorrhea.

Nowadays, although it's a rare herbalist who considers Our Lord's Candle as a cure for venereal disease, this old medicinal is still a source of a peerless shampoo, an excellent skin care lotion, and a fine leaf tea, rich in salicylic acid, which some arthritis victims claim relieves the pain, inflammation, and stiffness in their joints.

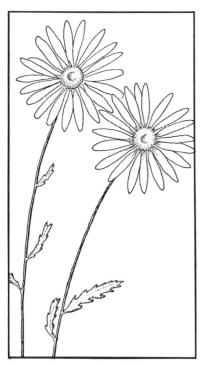

Ox-Eye Daisy

OX-EYE DAISY

Chrysanthaemum leucanthemum

Other names for the Ox-eye Daisy: Other common names for this plant are Field Daisy, Marguerite, Dog Daisy, Bull Daisy, White Weed, Poorland Daisy, Maudlin Daisy, Poverty Weed, and Moon Penny.

Where to find it: This perennial member of the Sunflower family (really a Chrysanthemum and not a true Daisy) is a native of the Old World now naturalized in America, and found in open spaces such as meadows, neglected parks, and other waste places. In California it's especially common in the central and northern parts of the state, as in Humboldt County where it grows alongside roadways in such profusion, so lushly and showily, it looks as if the residents planted it there to beautify the land.

How to know it when you see it: If you see lovely white Daisy-like flowers blooming abundantly in places like those described above and if their lower stem leaves are shaped rather like grapefruit spoons, complete with teeth, and their yellow heads are plump and prettily protruding, you've doubtless laid your eyes on the Ox-eye Daisy. If it appears to be growing like a weed, it's as it should be. *Chrysanthaemum leucanthemum* is a weed indeed, and though beloved to those who can't resist a pretty face, it's a bane and a bother to others.

Its lore. Since many herbals of the early nineteenth century still smacked of the influence of famous old-world healers like Nicholas Culpeper, some early settlers had been advocates of the Ox-eye Daisy long before they got to California. To those who believed in Culpeper, this plant was "a wound herb of good respect," a worthwhile treatment for ulcers and pustules, palsy, sciatica, and gout.

Through the years, the Ox-eye Daisy has served as an anti-spasmodic, a diuretic, a respected treatment for whooping cough and asthma, and as a soothing substitute for that better-known herb, Chamomile.

PENSTEMON

Penstemon spp.

Other names for the Penstemon: Some common names for various species of Penstemon are Hot Rock Penstemon, Foothill Penstemon, Showy Penstemon, and Royal Penstemon. The Cahuilla name for one species, the lovely Scarlet Bugler, was *Tuchilychungva*, a word meaning, literally, "hummingbird's kiss."

Where to find it: Many species of Penstemon are found growing in California, especially in the southern part of the state. Some are shrubs; some are herbs. Some are rather ungainly looking; some rank among the loveliest of all our wildflowers. Although a few, such as *P. anguineus*, can tolerate a moist habitat, most of these members of the Snapdragon family are found in dryer locations such as rocky crevices, limestone slopes, and gravelly or volcanic soils. The Cahuillas' beloved "hummingbird's kiss," better known as the Scarlet Bugler (*P. centranthifolius*), for example, thrives in dry disturbed places in southern California. The equally lovely Royal Penstemon, with its rose-red flowers and its bright green leaves, favors dry desert washes, and other disturbed locations at altitudes less than 6,000 feet.

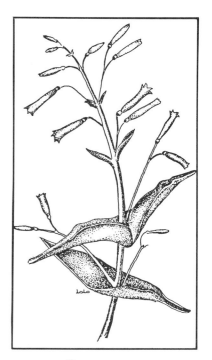

Penstemon

Its lore. After their Christianization, the Cahuilla Indians prized the "hummingbird's kiss" mainly as an ornamental plant, which they displayed at funerals and other church functions. Records are silent on the subject of its prior use as a medicine but it's probable, nonetheless, that the medicinal properties of this plant were well-known to these and other desert Indians as well as to the settlers who learned their ways.

Today a concoction made from this herb is used as a soothing application for the skin. Mashed and blended, it's sometimes mixed with other ingredients such as olive oil and used as a lotion for the treatment of rashes, cold sores, chapped hands, and other epidermal irritations.

PEONY

Paeonia brownii

Other names for the Peony: Two common names for this plant are Western Peony and California Peony

Where to find it: Often keeping company with Scrub Oak and Sagebrush, this wildflower can be found on dry slopes, in small meadows, in Yellow Pine forests, in chaparral country, and on foothill ridges at altitudes that range from 3,000 to 7,350 feet, in several California locations.

How to know it when you see it: Because of the way it droops as if it's too heavy for the stem that bears it, the dark, wine-colored flower of this native westerner sometimes goes unnoticed. The plant itself, which is often wider than it is tall, rarely reaches a height of one and a half feet, and its fleshy, bluish, unevenly dissected leaves often fail to draw attention to the hangdog flower. This unprepossessing Peony bears little resemblance to its cultivated kin.

Its lore. Several California Indian tribes, including the desert-dwelling Cahuillas, used the dried and powdered roots of this native western herb to concoct a variety of medicines with which they treated colds, sore throats, coughs, and chest congestion.

   In very small doses, Peony tea has been used for nervousness and melancholia and as a treatment for painful menstruation.

Comment: The consumption of even small amounts of this herb can cause nausea.

PIGWEED

Chenopodium californicum, C. fremontii, and *C. album*

Other names for the Pigweed: Other common names for the Pigweed are Lamb's Quarters, White Chenopodium, Goose-foot, and Careless Weed. To the Cahuilla Indians this plant was *Ki'awet.*

Where to find it: *C. californicum* is common on dry slopes and plains below 5,000 feet. *C. fremontii* likes dry places too, and is found in Pinyon-Juniper woods and Yellow Pine Forests at altitudes that range between 5,000 and 8,500 feet. *C. album* is a very common weed found almost anyplace where the soil is both rich and a bit neglected.

How to know it when you see it: In seeking *C. album,* which is possibly the most characteristic of the Pigweeds, look for a good-sized plant, up to seven feet tall, with a straight central stem, tiny, inconspicuous, ball-shaped flowers that appear in spikes, and leaves shaped like the footprints of geese. In spring its seeds are as green as the rest of the plant, but they begin to redden as fall comes on. The "album" in its name means white, and in this case refers to the unmistakable silvery sheen of its foliage. From a distance the leaves look as if they've been liberally sprayed with a can of silver paint.

Its lore. From the arid southern deserts to the moist and verdant northern lands, California Indians made good use of the various species of the common

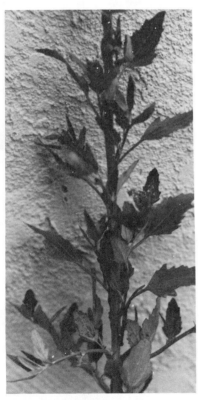

Pigweed

Pigweed, both as a food and as a medicine. While the Round Valley Indians were munching the cooked greens of the Pigweed, the Cahuillas were storing its grain in stashes fringing Coyote Canyon, one of their favorite haunts. And though these tribes were separated by many miles, and so can scarcely be said to have learned their healing arts one from the other, they both used Pigweed as a medicament for stomach problems. In the Round Valley it was the species *C. album* that healed the aching bellies of the Pomos or the Yukis or the Wailakis. On the desert it was *C. californicum* (which also yielded a useful soap) that served the same purpose for the innovative Cahuillas.

Some settlers made good use of Pigweed too, just as they had done back home in the eastern states, where Pigweed-leaf poultices had served to cure arthritis and rheumatism, while the juice from boiled greens had helped to soothe toothaches.

Like most bonafide weeds, Pigweed (so called because it's a favorite food of porcines) is considered a pest, and yet there's a sense in which it can be said to serve as a medicine for the earth itself, just as surely as it's served so many ailing humans. In truth, it feeds and enriches the soil where it's grown.

Comment: Since this is an herb which often contains toxic quantities of both oxalic acid and nitrate, it should be consumed in moderate amounts only.

PINE

Pinus spp.

Other names for various Pines: Whitebark Pine, Limber Pine, Western White Pine (also called Silver Pine), One-Leaved Pinyon, Ponderosa Pine, etc. The Cahuilla name for a Pine tree of any species was *Wexet*. The Little Lake name for the Ponderosa Pine, *Pinus ponderosa*, was *Cha-om*.

Where to find it: Since nearly one-fourth of all known species of the genus *Pinus* are richly represented in the state of California, and since one Pine or another is found growing at altitudes that range from sea level to 12,000 feet, it almost seems that it would be easier to list the locations where pine trees *aren't* found than those where they are. This isn't quite true, however. From the dwarfish, crooked-trunked Whitebark Pine (*P. albicaulis*), which is happiest where the air is rarified, to the famous lowland-dweller, the wind-ravaged Monterey Pine (*P. radiata*), it's safe to say that these native conifers favor dry slopes, rocky ridges, and gravelly bluffs, and that they aren't apt to be found where the soil is soggy.

How to know it when you see it: Since a Pine's cone is woodier and stiffer than those of other conifers, and its needles are borne in bundles held together by a paper-like sheath, it's not hard to tell a Pine tree from a Spruce or a Fir. The trick is in remembering all the characteristics that distinguish one Pine from another Pine. There are so many varieties of this evergreen species in California that when the famous traveler, David Douglas, wrote home about them in the 1800s, he feared that fellow naturalists might think he was "manufacturing pines" at his pleasure. Consider these, for example, to name just a few: The

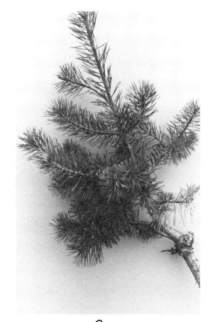

Pine

Whitebark Pine (*P. albicaulis*) is a homely tree, crooked-trunked and dwarfish; the common Sugar Pine (*P. Lambertiana*) is tall, well-formed, wide-spreading, a recognized beauty; the Bristlecone Pine (*P. aristata*) is bushy and massive; the Tamarack Pine (*P. Murrayan*) stands as tall and as straight as a telephone pole.

Its lore. All Pine trees, from the scraggliest of Desert Pinyons to the most imposing Ponderosa, were highly prized by the California Indians, some of whom heralded harvest time with fanfare and prayer. They looked to each specimen for all these things: the cones that contained the wonderfully edible nuts they savored; the needles they wove into the fabric of their baskets; the bark and pitch from which they made an assortment of salves, ointments, plasters, packs, creams, and teas; the wood they used for torches and kindling, or for the arduous "pain cooking" ceremony, wherein a shaman's healing prowess was intensified as she forced herself to remain at the side of a huge Pine fire and endure its stifling heat and smoke.

Cahuilla women used Pine pitch as a face cream to protect their skin from sunburn. To the Little Lakes the similar exudation of the Ponderosa served as a chewing gum and a medicine. Many tribes made a Pine-bark decoction to draw the soreness from burns and scalds, to stave off infection, to soothe and heal. Yet others swabbed sore throats with the pulverized dried resin, drank hot Pine-bark tea to treat their colds, or applied packs of warm pitch to bring boils to a head, draw out splinters, and ease away the aches of rheumatism, sciatica, and arthritis.

Today, Pine tea, said to be best when made from new pale-green needles in the spring, is still used by some herbalists, backpackers, hikers, and survivalists.

Comment: Although Pine tea is still drunk by some herb buffs and wild-food enthusiasts, the very needles from which it's made are reportedly toxic to livestock, especially in the winter months. So too are young Pine shoots. Although records are few, there are some known cases of Pine-needle poisoning and resultant abortion in California cattle who've chanced to browse on fallen trees, as they'll sometimes do even when good forage is available.

Pine toxin is destroyed by heat, which is apparently one reason why the tea has not proved harmful to human beings.

Note: For more information about teas made from species of *Pinus* and from other conifers as well, see "Digger Pine."

PINEAPPLE WEED

Matricaria matricarioides

Other names for the Pineapple Weed: This plant is also known as False Chamomile and Pineapple Chamomile.

Where to find it: This alien annual, probably introduced first to the eastern states, is an extremely common weed in waste places and disturbed spots all over California.

How to know it when you see it: Because of its small size (it rarely grows over a foot in height) and the familiar laciness of its pinnate leaves, this sweet-scented herb is often mistaken for wild Chamomile. Pineapple Weed is leafier, however, and its yellow-green flower cones are remarkably pineapple-shaped.

Its lore. Although the Pineapple Weed is not generally considered a medicinal herb, it's often been used as such for the simple reason that it's been mistaken for another species of *Matricaria*, the true Wild Chamomile, *M. chamomilla*. Furthermore, it's been given credit for the very same benefits that are commonly afforded by its well-known relative. This state of affairs could look like a full-blown case of the placebo effect if it weren't for the fact that the Cahuilla Indians once used this selfsame plant medicinally on the strength of its own virtues and not those of its kin. Ironically, the benefits reported by the Cahuillas, who had made no mistake in its use, were much the same as those reported by the misapprehenders. It settled their stomach. It cured their diarrhea. It soothed their colic.

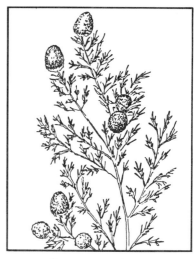

Pineapple Weed

PLANTAIN

Plantago spp.

Other names for the Plantain: Depending on the species, Plantain plants are known as Cuckoo's Bread, Ribgrass, Way-Bread, Cribworth, Buckhorn, Ripple Grass, Devil's Shoestring, Snakeweed, and Soldiers' Herb.

Where to find it: Plantain is one of our most familiar weeds, a perennial that grows not only all over California but all over the world. Here it's such a common herb it can be found in almost any moist and open place; from dooryard to meadow, from streamside to park lawn.

How to know it when you see it: From the homely little lawn-hugging types that gardeners bemoan to the lush *Plantago major* that looks as if it's escaped from a tropical jungle, there's a great variation between one species of Plantain and another. Yet they do have common characteristics that render identification fairly easy. Their leaves are always entirely basal, outward-flaring, very fibrous, and lined with parallel veins. The flowers that tip their slender stalks are tiny, nondescript, and inconspicuous. When they're crushed or broken, the leaves of the Plantain feel slippery to the touch, as if they've been dipped in the whites of eggs.

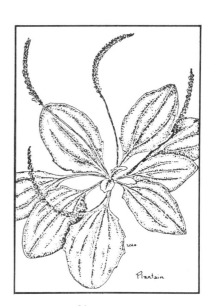

Plantain

Its lore. This is one of those beautifully versatile herbs that served the settlers as well as it did the native Americans who peopled this land before them, a fact as true in California as it was in the eastern states. (There it was the source of several popular remedies, and the purported treatment for ailments that ranged from snakebite to syphilis.) Many of the Shoshones, including, most probably, California's Kosho or Panamint Indians, used the fibrous leaves of Plantain plants as a wet dressing for their wounds and sores. Settlers and Indians alike made Plantain poultices, which they applied externally for the treatment of abraded skin, general itching, arthritis, sprains, gout, intestinal parasites, and all sorts of poisonous bites. Plantain tea, taken internally, was considered good for skin ailments, faulty menstruation, nasal congestion, minor intestinal upset, fevers, and general debility, while the seeds of the plant, so similar to psyllium, were used as a laxative.

No longer extolled as a cure for snakebite or venereal disease, Plantain is still considered a useful medicinal plant and is a hiker's favorite backpack remedy for that plague of the wilderness, the common mosquito bite.

POISON OAK

Toxicodendron diversilobum (formerly *Rhus diversiloba*)

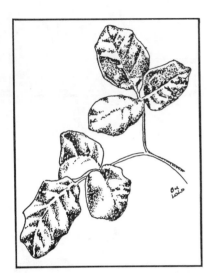

Poison Oak.

Other names for Poison Oak: This plant is sometimes called Poison Sumac or Fire Oak. The Wailaki name for Poison Oak was *Kots-ta.* To the Pomo it was *Ma-tu-ya-ho.* To the Spanish Californios it was known as *Yedra.*

Where to find it: This much-detested member of the Sumac family has a preference for low places such as moist thickets, coastal scrub lands, and wooded slopes and foothills at altitudes below 5,000 feet. Look for it by the sides of streams, in shady groves of Oaks, or in the underlayer of the tall forest. In woodlands it's apt to be found fraternizing with more beneficent plants such as Hazelnut, Huckleberry, Rhododendron, Dogwood, Oregon Grape, and Wax Myrtle. It's not hard to find this plant; in fact, it's hard to stay clear of it. It's one of the most widespread wildings in the state.

How to know it when you see it: The leaves of this highly poisonous plant—a showy crimson in both spring and fall—are trifoliate, lobed, and sometimes toothed. They're not always easy to identify, however. To trick and deceive seems to be their nature. Sometimes they have a sheen like a fine patina; sometimes their surface is matte and dull. To add further confusion, they vary in size. In fact, variation is the mode of the entire plant; sometimes it's a shrub; sometimes it's an earth-hugging vine, sometimes it winds around trees and hangs from *their* branches, where (to the detriment of the passerby who reaches up and aimlessly plucks off a leaf) it poses as their own foliage.

The fruit of the Poison Oak is a small poisonous berry, whitish in color, as are its flowers.

Its lore. When translated, the Pomo name for this plant means "the southern fire doctor." This is an interesting commentary on a species that some writers aver was never poisonous at all to the full-blooded native Californian. If it wasn't poisonous to them then why did the Pomos call it "fire doctor?" Were they reflecting only upon the woes it spelled for the white man? Or is it as some other observers have noted? Were Indians exempt from the hazardous effects of Poison Oak only *after* they'd somehow rendered themselves immune? Was this a feat they accomplished by drinking small quantities of Poison Oak tea, as was once reported of the desert Cahuillas? Or was it, as others have suggested, that the California Indians ate a green sprig of the plant every springtime and thereby protected themselves for the rest of the year?

We may never know the answers to these questions. This much is a certainty, however; this well-known plant—a bane to outdoor folk nowadays—was once a boon to many an Indian. To the Pomos, who used its slender stems in the construction of their beautiful baskets and its juice as a good black dye with which to color them, it was a highly effective wart remover and a cure for ring-worm. For the Wailakis, the fresh leaves of the plant (if applied hastily enough) could conteract the deadly venom of the rattlesnake.

Comment: According to statistics, seven out of ten people in the country can develop a sensitivity to this extremely hazardous plant, which, except for its pollen, is highly toxic in every part. Dermatitis usually develops between 24 and 72 hours after contact with the plant itself, or sometimes with *anything,* including clothing and pets, that may have happened to brush up against it. Droplets of the juice of Poison Oak can even spread in the air by way of the smoke from burning stems and leaves. Individuals who are particularly sensitive to its powerful toxin, urushiol, may react in less than 24 hours and may experience symptoms such as swelling of the throat and eyes, nausea, cramps, vomiting, and diarrhea, in addition to the usual itching rash.

There is nothing to indicate that victims will become immune to urushiol after the first occasion of exposure. On the contrary, symptoms sometimes worsen with each new contact. Do not tamper with this plant.

PRICKLY POPPY

Argemone spp.

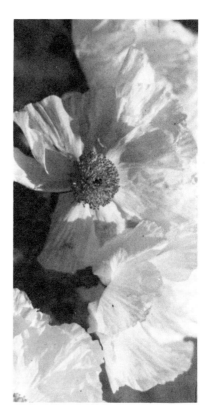

Prickly Poppy

Other names for the Prickly Poppy: This plant is sometimes called Thistle Poppy or Mexican Poppy. The Spanish name for the plant is *Cardo Santo.*

Where to find it: One species of Prickly Poppy, *A. corymbosa,* is a true south-westerner. Dwelling on dry slopes, flats, and high plateaus, in Creosote Bush scrub, in the Mojave Desert, and other arid regions where it blooms from April through May, it's found at altitudes that range from 1,400 to 3,500 feet. *A. munita,* another moisture-shirker, abides in chaparral country and in the coast ranges from San Luis Obispo County to lower California, occasionally in altitudes up to 6,000 feet.

How to know it when you see it: Look for a plant from two to five feet tall that is such a remarkable study in contradiction you'll think you've been fooled by your eyes when you spot it. Its breathtakingly lovely Poppy-like flower has six great showy petals that appear to be made from tissue paper. Crepy and delicate-looking, contrasting beautifully with their golden-yellow centers, these petals seem to bear no relation whatever to the barbed and stickery bluish-green leaves that poke upward ominously beneath them.

Most people are so captivated by the Prickly Poppy's papery bloom that they long to pick it, to press it, to keep it with them as a memento long after they've departed its arid homeland. Few people do so, however. The lethal-looking foliage, so much like that of the most pernicious thistle, precludes the picking and pulling to all but those who've donned their leather gloves. Hence, the plant usually remains intact until the flowers lose their petals, one at a time, from natural causes.

Its lore. Named for a Poppy-like flower that was used as an eye medicine in the days of Pliny, this plant's generic title means "cataract of the eye." Ironically, in our own country, though not in California, some Indian tribes have used an extract of this plant's armored leaves for the treatment of the same organ, the human eye. It's a dangerous use, however, and one that's distinctly out of favor. Even in the past, Prickly Poppy was usually employed only in a highly diluted form (its acrid yellow juices mixed with about five or six parts water), for the external treatment of hives and rashes and other skin ailments. Nowadays, the herb has fallen into almost complete disuse, as well it should have, in the light of its extreme toxicity.

Warning: Prickly Poppy plants contain several toxic alkaloids. Poisoning has occurred when grain has become accidentally contaminated with *Argemone* seeds or when people have incautiously experimented with the herb. Symptoms include diarrhea, vomiting, visual problems, fainting, and coma.

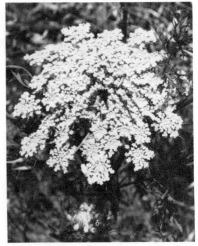

Queen Anne's Lace

QUEEN ANNE'S LACE

Daucus carota

Other names for Queen Anne's Lace: This common, medicinal plant is also known as Bird's-nest, the Bird's Nest Weed, Crow's-nest, Wild Carrot, and Devil's Plague.

Where to find it: A biennial plant that hails from Europe, Queen Anne's Lace is found growing profusely in meadows, on roadsides, in vacant lots, and in pasture lands, especially in California.

How to know it when you see it: The popular name of this alien weed serves as its best possible description. The flat-topped umbels of clustered white flowers—as many as 500 of them—that grace its willowy, branching stems are as lacy-looking as the doilies that a queen might place beneath her favorite vases. And in the center of each of these, like a secret symbol, there nestles the single blood-red flower that inspired the legend that surrounds this plant. (It's said that when the good Queen Anne pricked her finger as she was doing her dainty needlework, a drop of her royal blood landed on that single center stitch to leave its mark forever.)

Another of the plant's popular monikers also serves as a good description of *Daucus carota.* As they age, the lacy umbels begin to dry and fold upward in such a way that they bear a marked resemblance to the nests of some songbirds.

Yet a third name, "Wild Carrot," affords another distinguishing feature of this medicinal weed, which after all, truly *is* a carrot in the rough. Its root smells just like that of the familiar garden vegetable.

The leaves of Queen Anne's Lace are arranged alternately on their rather hairy stems and are pinnately divided. Other than the blood-red center, the umbels of flowers are generally white, occasionally roseate, or soft, pale yellow. The plant reaches a height of three feet.

Its lore. There never was a weed more weedy, more insistent on growing in the places that it chooses, more stubborn and pesky than that legendary old European, Queen Anne's Lace, really nothing more and nothing less than a wild carrot, and wild in every sense of the word. Yet, paradoxically, there are few weeds more beautiful and more wrapped in legend, nor many better reputed as a stand-by remedy for common flatulence (gas on the stomach).

This herb, once believed a preventive medicine to ward off epileptic seizures, was also used as a diuretic and a treatment for kidney stones.

Queen Anne's Lace is currently enjoying a comeback, not so much for its purported medicinal properties, which have never been substantiated, as for its tasty first-year roots, a favorite of survivalists and wild-food enthusiasts who find them as delicious as cultivated carrots fresh-picked from the garden.

Caution: Care must be taken not to confuse Queen Anne's Lace with several very dangerous umbel-bearing plants such as Poison Hemlock (*Conium maculatum*) to which it bears some resemblance.

REDBUD

Cercis occidentalis

Other names for the Redbud: Another popular English name for this plant is Judas Tree. The Concow had two names for the Redbud, *Dop* and *Tal'k*. The Yokia called it *Ka-la a ka-la*. To the Yuki it was *Cha-a;* to the Little Lake, *Mu-la*.

Where to find it: The Redbud favors canyons, dry slopes, coastal ranges, arid flats, and foothills at altitudes below 3,500 feet.

How to know it when you see it: Rounded or spreading in shape, the Redbud is usually a shrub but sometimes a small tree that reaches a height of twenty feet. Its smooth-margined and heart-shaped leaves are round or notched at the apex, and two to four inches in width. Its pods are dull red, its flowers, which appear in the spring before the leaves do, are a lovely lavender-red.

Its lore. Details about the early medicinal use of the beautiful Redbud are sketchy at best, but of such interest, even so, that they can't go unmentioned. In the old days, some of California's early settlers, especially those who dwelt in northern California's secluded Round Valley, used the bark of this lovely native plant as a substitute for Quinine. With their homemade Redbud remedy they treated their aching bodies, their chills and their fevers.

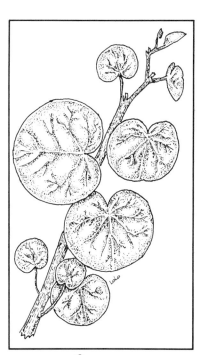

Redbud

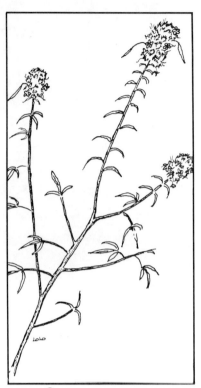

Rocky Mountain
Bee Plant

ROCKY MOUNTAIN BEE PLANT

Cleome serrulata

Other names for the Rocky Mountain Bee Plant: This plant is also known as Stinkweed, Spiderflower, Bee Plant, and Mountain Bee's Plant.

Where to find it: Found throughout the west, the Rocky Mountain Bee Plant is happiest in sagebrush areas, on plains and rangelands, in open woodlands, and on mountain slopes and hillsides. In some places (as in the Owens Valley, where the atmosphere sometimes seems similar only to the innards of an oven), it grows so abundantly as to form walls of color for the roadways there.

How to know it when you see it: Look for a tall-stemmed, multi-branched plant with top-heavy spikes of long-blooming flowers, each of which bears four sepals and four petals, and a distinctly-visible claw. These blooms, showy enough to grace a wildflower garden, vary greatly in color. Some are yellow; some are purple; some are rose-tinted, or white. Whatever their hue, wherever they grow—as their name implies—the Rocky Mountain Bee Plants are frequented by nectar-seeking insects.

Its lore. Considering how beloved it is to the bees, it's not surprising that *Cleome serrulata* was once cultivated as a honey plant. The surprise lies rather in the fact that the bees who visited it were not nearly as productive as had been expected. Actually this sort of "has-been" status seems to be the plight of this once-popular annual. It used to be a folk remedy too, a treatment for such diverse conditions as anemia, stomach complaints, and insect bites; now its medicinal properties, as forgotten as its honey to all but the bees, whose stings (ironically) it once soothed, aren't even mentioned in most current herbals. Yet once, Californians used it to cure their ills; that's a fact that negligence cannot erase.

Comment: Because of an accumulation of free nitrates, this plant can be harmful to cattle.

SAGE

Salvia spp.

Other names for Sage: Popular names of various species of this plant are Chia, Crimson Sage, Purple Sage, White Sage, Thistle Sage, Blue Sage, Black Sage and others. To the Numlaki Indians, Chia (*Salvia columbariae*) was known as *Clu-po*. The Cahuilla Indians called this same plant *Pasal*. The Cahuilla name for Thistle Sage (*S. carduacea*) was *Palnat*, whereas both White Sage and Black Sage were known to them as *Qas'ily*.

Where to find it: From one border of the state to another, you'll find some kind of Sage growing almost everywhere in California, but look to the south for the largest stands as well as the biggest variety of types and sizes.

Chia (*Salvia columbariae*) is common in dry open places, especially where the soil has been disturbed. You'll find it thriving in Creosote Bush scrub, in chaparral, and in foothill woods, at altitudes usually below 4,000 feet, but occasionally as high as 7,000 feet. Thistle Sage (*S. carduacea*) likes gravelly places below 4,500 feet. White Sage (*S. apiana*) is common on dry benches and slopes, as is Black Sage (*S. mellifera*), but whereas the former will flourish at altitudes up to 5,000 feet, the latter is happier in low-lying places.

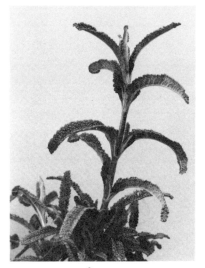

Sage

How to know it when you see it: Some *Salvia* plants are herbs, some are shrubs, almost all are strongly aromatic, square-stemmed, and bear opposite leaves. The flowers, pink, red, blue, purple or even white, depending on the species, are usually whorled and arranged in spikes, racemes, or panicles. The seeds are nutlets, small and smooth.

Chia, a very common and wide-ranging Sage that was highly prized by the native Californians, boasts roundish clusters of tiny, purple, two-lipped flowers, arranged on the top of their stems, rather like the balls on batons. Its leaves, unlike those of most *Salvia* plants, are semi-pinnately lobed, and rather lace-like in appearance.

Another favorite of the desert tribes, the White Sage, which blooms from April to July, is scrubby below, has lance-shaped leaves that are crowded at the base, and bears white flowers that generally boast some trace of lavender.

Its lore. Chia is one of those wild medicinal plants so esteemed by the Indians that the early Spanish settlers, watching them use it, taking note of the cures it wrought, and how quickly it wrought them, began to see that here was a herb that could serve them well too, one that surely rated a corner in their medicine cabinets. That's where they put it, and that's where it stayed for many a year, just as it also stayed in their pantries to serve as a food, as tasty to them as it was to the natives. By 1849, Chia seeds were selling in Los Angeles stores for as much as eight dollars a pound. To say that they were well worth the price, in the eyes of those early Californios, is a double entendre, for that was one special medicinal use of this nineteenth century wonder plant: a cure for eye inflammation. Just a couple of seeds placed under the lid at bedtime and in the morning all redness was gone; the orb was clear as a babe's. These costly seeds had other uses too, of course, including a good old-fashioned "Indian Poultice" of Chia mush, a stand-by application for boils and ulcers and slow-to-heal sores.

White Sage served the same purposes for the Indians as Chia did, and a few others besides. Its seeds were both a food and an eye cleanser, but it was the versatile leaves that boasted the longest list of medicinal uses. As a treatment for the common cold, they were smoked, eaten, and inhaled in the sweathouse. Crushed and mixed with water they were used as a shampoo, a hair color, and a straightener. Mashed and likewise mixed with liquid, they served as an underarm deodorant.

As both culinary and medicinal herbs, all of the aromatic Sages still rank high with California's herb buffs, survivalists, and wild-food enthusiasts alike. Sage tea, once believed to cure palsy and make men wise, is used as a refreshing beverage, a general pick-me-up, a treatment for laryngitis, a stomach tonic, and a remedy for excess bodily secretions of every variety. Modern herbalists deem it one of the best herbs available for decreasing the lactation of either woman or beast when it's time for weaning.

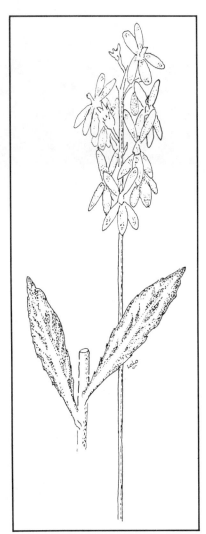

Scarlet Lobelia

SCARLET LOBELIA

Lobelia cardinalis

Other names for the Scarlet Lobelia: This plant is also known as Cardinal Flower, Red Lobelia, and Eyebright.

Where to find it: Not a common plant, the beautiful Scarlet Lobelia thrives in shady places where the soil is rich, moist, or truly wet, along the edges of streams, in bogs, in meadows and in low, damp woodlands at altitudes up to 6,000 feet, in southern California.

How to know it when you see it: If you see hummingbirds hovering over a lovely, upright, red-flowered plant in a damp and shady place somewhere in southern California, you may have stumbled on the Scarlet Lobelia. It's an eye-catching plant to people as well as to birds. Ranging in height from three to six feet, it boasts lancelike leaves, and showy two-lipped flowers arranged in terminal clusters.

Its lore. Records of Indian usage of this plant are scanty, but it's known that its leaves were smoked for medicinal purposes by several tribes. Occasionally settlers followed suit, especially victims of bronchial problems, for the herb was a specific cure for conditions like theirs. Sometimes they were healed; sometimes they were poisoned. Although it's not as potent as the much more controversial *Lobelia inflata* to which it's related, Scarlet Lobelia is not to be trifled with. Even those herbalists who praise it highly are careful to point out the dangers of overdose.

Warning: When green, the entire Lobelia plant is toxic, less so when dried. Symptoms of poisoning are dry throat, nausea, headache, vertigo, exhaustion, constriction of pupils, convulsions, respiratory failure, and coma. Deaths have occurred through overdose and misuse of some species of the genus.

SHEPHERD'S PURSE

Capsella bursa-pastoris

Other names for the Shepherd's Purse: This homely old medicinal herb is also known as Mother's Heart, Shovelweed, Caseweed, Cocowort, Shepherd's Heart, Toywort, and Pickpocket. One of its most commonly-used Spanish names is *Bolsa de Pastor*.

Where to find it: A lover of waste places, especially those that are loamy or sandy and much visited by the sun, Shepherd's Purse can be found throughout the state in such spots as pastures, lawns, schoolyards, gardens, and vacant lots, at altitudes up to 7,000 feet.

How to know it when you see it: Many of the popular names of this common weed are highly descriptive of its most distinguishing feature, its smooth, brownish seed pods, which are purse-shaped, or heart-shaped, or shovel-shaped, depending upon the eye of the beholder. As to its other features which are somewhat variable, it can grow as tall as eighteen inches; it bears tiny, in-conspicuous white flowers; its stem rises from a rosette of lobed or divided basal leaves.

Its lore. Though it was a foreigner in the land, the Cahuilla Indians adopted this long-time favorite of the European herbalists and added it to their own compendium of trusted remedies. They found that a cup of Shepherd's Purse tea was good medicine for a case of dysentery.

Early settlers, who had even a smattering of knowledge about herbs, knew this plant well. Weed though it was, they were delighted to find it thriving in California. Long reputed as an herb that could halt excessive bleeding, it was a useful wilding to have around in a time and place where the hazards were many, injuries were frequent, and the nearest doctor was sometimes more than a day away.

Homemade ointments, salves, teas, and decoctions made from Shepherd's Purse are still sometimes used today, especially for such conditions as hemor-rhoids, excessive menstruation, nosebleed, and cuts.

SNEEZEWEED

Helenium spp.

Other names for the Sneezeweed: The Pomo Indian name for this plant was *Ka-pa sho-pa*. To the Yokia it was *Kot-ka-yachdo*.

Where to find it: Most species of Sneezeweed are distinct moisture lovers apt to be found in marshes, damp meadows, on wet slopes, and by the sides of streams.

As John Woodhouse Audubon noted in his 1850 journal, this plant was once particularly abundant near the town of Coloma, the little settlement where gold was first discovered at Sutter's famous mill. "'Sutter's Mills' is about fifty miles, nearly east of Sacramento," he wrote. "The road to it after passing the first four or five miles runs through a sandy soil, covered at present with what we call 'sneezeweed'."

How to know it when you see it: Members of the Sunflower family, the various Sneezeweeds found in California are yellow-flowered annual or perennial herbs, with alternate leaves and simple or branched stems, and range in height

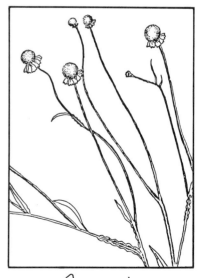

Sneezeweed

from one to five feet. The flower heads of most *Helenium* plants are roundish, comparatively large and conspicuous, sometimes almost hiding the white rays which are often relaxed downward, lending the flower an almost wilted appearance. The leaves of Bigelow's Sneezeweed (*H. bigelovi*) appear to be a continuation of the stems—or vice versa—so that the latter look "leafy-edged," as if they bear ruffles. This same species bears solitary, yellow, ball-like flower heads.

Its lore. That Sneezeweed was never a widely-used herb is not altogether surprising; the plant is acrid-tasting, hotter than red peppers, stronger than whiskey, and sometimes, as in the case of *H. hoopesii*, toxic to livestock, if not to humankind. Nonetheless, in one locality, at least, it was once considered an important medicinal plant. To the Indians of Round Valley it was almost a specific for treating venereal complaints, a use that was surely bound to lend it status.

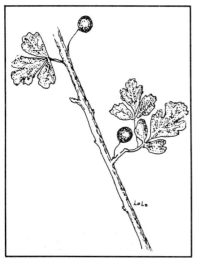

Squaw Bush

SQUAW BUSH

Rhus trilobata

Other names for the Squaw Bush: To the Yokia Indians this plant was known as *Bo-bo-e*. To the Cahuilla it was *Selet*.

Where to find it: Squaw Bush is common in canyons and washes, in coastal sage scrub, and in foothill woods, usually at altitudes below 3,500 feet. Look for it too in chaparral, where you may find it consorting with Manzanita, Redberry, and small Live Oaks, not to mention its ill-reputed look-alike kin, Poison Oak.

How to know it when you see it: Squaw Bush is a small deciduous shrub, from two to five feet in height, that happens to look a lot like its infamous relative, the much-detested Poison Oak. Its aromatic trifoliate leaves bear a terminal three-lobed leaflet and two lateral leaflets, which are almost oval; its branches are spreading, sometimes slightly drooping; its tiny flowers, which bloom from March to April before the new leaves appear, are pale yellow; its fruit is a fleshy red berry.

Its lore. Prized by some California Indians for its wood, from which they used to fashion seed beaters, by some for its lemony-tasting berries, by yet others for its twigs, which were woven into baskets and mats, the Squaw Bush also had a role to play in the folk medicine of early California. To the Cahuilla, the fruit of the Squaw Bush, which they also savored as a food, was the source of a restorative tonic for the stomach. To the Yokia, these same berries, dried and pulverized, served either as a medicinal powder or as the prime ingredient in a lotion, both of which were used in the treatment of the smallpox that once raged with such a fury through the northern lands they loved.

STORKBILL

Erodium cicutarium

Other names for the Storkbill: This little medicinal plant is also known as Fila-ree and Heron's Bill. Its Spanish name is *Alfilerillo*.

Where to find it: This small weed, a native of the Mediterranean, is common from one end of California to the other, in dry places, at altitudes less than 6,000 feet.

How to know it when you see it: A member of the Geranium family, Storkbill is one of the easiest to identify of all medicinal weeds. Its stems, which are borne in prostrate rosettes, are red and hairy; its flowers are five-petaled, deli-cate, and a lovely shade of rose; its taproot is turnip-like; its leaves are finely-divided and lobed; and its seeds are long beaks—shaped very much like the bills of storks.

Its lore. It's believed that this plant was introduced into California by the early Spanish settlers and that it's been used medicinally ever since. A mild herb and generally considered safe to use in either tea or poultice form, it's been em-ployed as a treatment for water retention, and for gout and rheumatism. Com-mon as it is, it's a pretty little plant and makes an excellent potherb.

SWEET CLOVER

Melilotus spp.

Other names for the Sweet Clover: Other English names for this plant are King's Clover, Sweet Lucerne, Melilot, Yellow Sweet-Clover, and White Sweet Clover. Its Spanish name is *Alfalfon*.

Where to find it: A native of Eurasia, Sweet Clover is found in disturbed places in many California locations. The yellow-flowered *Melilotus officinalis*, is an un-common California resident found occasionally in fields, on roadsides, and in other waste places. The much more common White Sweet Clover, *M. albus*, is abundant in damp waste places, especially in southern California. Another species, *M. indicus*, is a low-land lover seen growing in waste places all over the state.

How to know it when you see it: Averaging from three to five feet in height, this herb bears spikelike racemes of many small pea-like flowers, palmate leaf-lets, and an odor so sweet that no foraging creature can resist it.

Its lore. The Clover-loving California Indians must surely have adopted this vanilla-scented alien as a food, just as they did another foreigner, the Burr Clo-ver, which quickly became a favorite of theirs. But when it came to its medicinal usage, Sweet Clover was not the province of native Californians, but rather

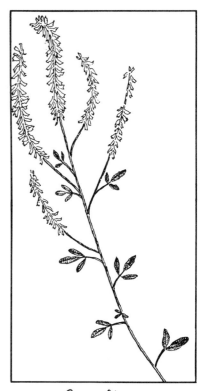

Sweet Clover

that of the latter-day residents, people whose folk medicine had always included this much-beloved herb.

Historically, a tea made from Sweet Clover has been used to soothe stomachaches, to relieve flatulence, and to ease the symptoms of intestinal disturbances of every variety. Externally it's been applied in the form of poultices for the treatment of sore breasts, aching joints, swelling and inflammation. Happily, Sweet Clover is still in good repute today.

Warning: When this herb rots and ferments, it becomes an anticoagulant. Its consumption, therefore, can cause internal hemorrhaging in animals and humans. The plant is harmless in its fresh state.

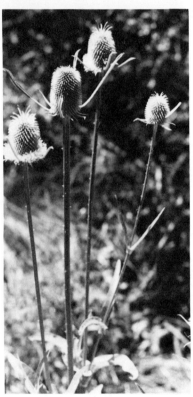

Teasel

TEASEL

Dipsacus spp.

Other names for the Teasel: This plant is also known as Venus' Basin, Wild Teasel, Water Thistle, and Kitchen Sink Plant.

Where to find it: This prickly biennial from Eurasia is naturalized now in California and is seen growing wild in ditches, old fields, and other wastelands.

How to know it when you see it: Described at once as prickly, bristly, and spiny, the Teasel is as easy to identify as a plant could possibly be. Its lance-shaped leaves, bearing their own set of stickers, are paired and fused at their bases in such a way as to lend them a wrap-around effect. Prickly too are the stout stems, which bear tiny, tubular, lavender-blue flowers, tightly packed in bristly flowerheads that boast literally hundreds of tiny hooked spikes, all of which are surrounded, fittingly enough, by spiny bracts. A unique feature of the plant's structure is a little water-tight basin at the juncture of the two upper leaves, where a pool forms whenever it rains.

Its lore. Nowadays the Teasel is best known for its big, showy seedheads that are often used in dry flower arrangements, bouquets, and centerpieces. But in times past, California's rural residents used the plant for dozens of practical purposes, for example, brushing their clothing, picking lint, carding wool, and the like. There was plenty of precedent for this sort of usage, for this is the plant that the Romans employed, centuries ago, to "tease" the nap of their fine woolen fabric, and it was used commercially in much the same manner right here in the United States for many years. But in the realm of California folk medicine, the fascinating Teasel had always fallen short of the reputation it held in other places and other times. Once it was a much-respected remedy: its root was mixed with wine and applied to fistulas and warts and skin inflammations of various types. And a favorite prescription of old-country herbalists—a cure they perceived as nature's own eye lotion—was the rainwater that collected in the Teasel's natural basin, that little pool at the juncture of the plant's fused upper leaves.

TOYON

Heteromeles arbutifolia

Other names for the Toyon: Other English names for this plant are Christmas Berry and California Christmas Berry. The Pomo Indians called it *But-za-za*. The Yokia called it *Ki-yi*, while to the Yuki it was *Mil-ko-che*.

Where to find it: The Toyon is a common tree-like shrub that is at home on semi-arid slopes, in foothill woods, and in chaparral communities where it sometimes fraternized with such plants as Flannel Bush, Chamise, Coffeeberry, Mountain Mahogany, and Scrub Oak. This handsome shrub is found throughout most of California at altitudes below 4,000 feet.

How to know it when you see it: Distinguished especially by its big clusters of red berries, appropriately conspicuous in the month of December and thereby lending it a holly-like appearance, this freely-branching evergreen grows to heights that range between ten and twenty-five feet. It's further characterized by its very rigid and prominently serrated leaves, which are elliptical to oblong in shape.

Its lore. Since it's been used so often to "deck the halls" at Christmas time, the fame of the decorative Toyon tree has always been more associated with holiday cheer than it has with aches and pains and remedies. Nonetheless, to the Pomo Indians, the Yukis, and the Yokias, who also prized the plant for its edible fruit, the bark and the leaves of the Toyon once made an effective decoction for treating stomach-aches, including, no doubt, those they got from eating too many Toyon berries!

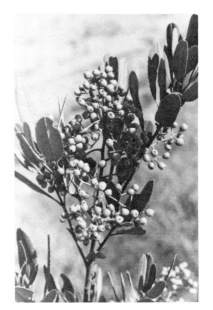

Toyon

TURKEY MULLEIN

Eremocarpus setigerus

Other names for the Turkey Mullein: Two other popular names for this plant are Dove Weed and Fish Locoweed. The Yuki name for the Turkey Mullein was *Ke-chil wa-e-mok*. The Pomo called it *Sha um*. Its Spanish names is *Yerba del pescado*.

Where to find it: Drawn to sandy soil and dry places, this exceedingly common native weed is found in coastal scrub, in foothill woods, in grasslands, on desert edges, and probably most often of all on the shoulders of backroads and freeways over much of the state.

How to know it when you see it: The sweet-smelling Turkey Mullein grows low to the ground (from one to eight inches high) in compact, mound-shaped, velvety gray rosettes, as neat and trim-looking as if they're regularly tended by some dedicated gardener.

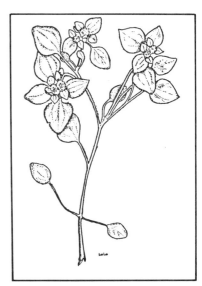

Turkey Mullein

Its lore. Beloved to wild Mourning Doves, who announce its presence with their melancholy coos, dear to the turkey—by which fact it earned its popular moniker—this abundantly-growing plant was once also greatly prized by certain tribes of California Indians, as well as some of the Spanish settlers who followed their example. They called it "fish soaproot," and used its bruised leaves as a poison to stupefy fish and make them easier to catch. And some Indians, especially the Concows, used the plant medicinally. The selfsame leaves that sedated the fish served as the source of three stand-by remedies deemed powerful enough for serious ailments like chest disorders and typhoid fever. One of these was a poultice, which was applied to the chest; one was a decoction with which to wash the feverish body; the third was a weak infusion, taken internally for the treatment of chills and fevers. Some settlers, observing the Concow cures, also made medicinal use of this strong-smelling herb, though probably only for a decade or two.

Warning: Cattle have suffered diarrhea from eating large quantities of Turkey Mullein, and there is at least one known case in which geese have died from consumption of the plant.

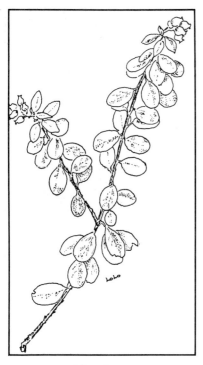

Uva-Ursi

UVA-URSI

Arctostaphylos uva-ursi

Other names for Uva-Ursi: This plant is also known as Kinnikinnick, Bearberry, Sandberry, Mealberry, Red Bearberry, Bear's Grape, Bear's Billberry, Upland Cranberry, Hog Cranberry, and Creeping Manzanita. Its Spanish name is *Coralillo*.

Where to find it: This perennial evergreen, found at elevations all the way up to 10,000 feet, is a limestone lover, most at home where the soil is poor and sandy, gravelly and coarse.

How to know it when you see it: With its bark the color of burgundy wine, Uva-Ursi is an attractive, creeping shrub, an earth-hugging member of the heath family that grows in a thick carpet in its favorite habitats. Its ovate leaves are a lively green that darken and toughen with time, and ultimately get so leathery they look like shoemakers' castaways. Its flowers, which are replaced in August by orange-red berries, are bell-shaped and misty pink.

Its lore. Like the burly mountain men who roved the wilderness with legendary verve, the Indians used the bitter-tasting leaves of the Uva-Ursi when they were miles between springs, streams, or water holes and their throats were thirsty and parched. One hearty chomp or two and the saliva would begin to flow again.

But to these earliest rovers of California, as well as to all of those who followed in their footsteps, Uva-Ursi was far more than a thirst reliever. It was a healer too, a remedy for ailments that ranged from bronchitis to bedwetting. Self-styled herbalists took it internally, generally in the form of a well-steeped leaf tea, for the general health of the reproductive system, for kidney stones, for menstrual problems, for bladder infections, for gleet, for catarrh, and for the hemorrhaging that sometimes followed childbirth. Occasionally the leaves were steeped in rum or brandy or whiskey instead of water, and the resulting tonic "tea" was highly extolled by some (to the tune of hiccoughs, no doubt) for its phenomenal healing prowess. Externally, both types of Uva-Ursi tea were applied to relieve the pain of sprains and bruises, as an antiseptic for sores and cuts, and as a soothing lotion for the awful itch of Poison Oak.

Warning: It is believed that large doses of Uva-Ursi can be toxic.

WAKE ROBIN

Trillium spp.

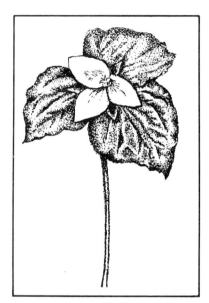

Wake Robin

Other names for the Wake Robin: This plant is also known as Trillium, Birthroot, Indian Shamrock, Indian Balm, Ground Lily, and Three-leaved Nightshade. The Little Lake Indians called it *Ki-ka-he-um*. To the Wailaki it was *Be-cha-te-chu*, while to the Yuki it was *Zhal-zhoi-e*.

Where to find it: This lovely plant is most often found in moist, shady woodland spots, where it sometimes keeps company with other woods dwellers like Buttercups and Violets and the deep green Wild Ginger with its heart-shaped leaves. Sometimes, as in northern California where it's so much at home, little companies of *Trillium* are seen growing right at the foot of tall conifers. The author recalls seeing one particularly lovely specimen that had sprouted up so close to a towering Mendocino giant that it appeared to be growing out of the tree instead of the soil around it.

Giant Trillium (*T. chloropetalum*) is found in brushy or wooded slopes at altitudes generally below 3,500 feet. Coast Trillium (*T. ovatum*) seeks moist wooded slopes in Redwood and mixed evergreen forests. *T. rivile* prefers rocky stream banks in Yellow Pine forests in Del Norte and Siskiyou counties.

How to know it when you see it: A child's typical description of the Wake Robin—"a pretty plant with a merry-go-round of three big leaves and just one pretty flower to ride on it"—is almost enough to identify this remarkable member of the Lily family. The Giant Trillium bears three great broadly oval leaves that are a strangely-mottled purple and appear somehow purposefully marked—as with some secret hieroglyphs (left by a wood nymph perhaps) yet to be deciphered. A variation of this species, *T. giganteum*, which was the Wake Robin best-known to the Yuki and the Wailaki Indians, grows to a height of twenty-one inches, has a stout stem, bears a whorl of round to ovate leaves that are broader than they are long, and boasts a flower that is deep red to lilac. The flowers of *T. rivile* are sometimes clear white, sometimes marked with rose-carmine. Unlike these other Trillium plants, whose single blooms appear at the juncture where the three leaves meet, yet another species, *T. ovatum*, bears its deep rose-colored flower atop a long slim pedicel that rises up above its three sharp-pointed green leaves like a miniature flagpole.

Its lore. In centuries past, The Yukis and Wailakis were as extravagant in their praise of the medicinal prowess of this native American plant as most Californians today are of its unsurpassed beauty. As those Indians told the naturalist V. K. Chestnut, who so avidly studied the lore of the northern tribes in the late 1800s, the Wake Robin was simply "good for any kind of sick."

Elsewhere in America, the Indians, as well as the settlers who followed their ways, used concoctions made from the tubers of this lovely plant as a general tonic, as a treatment for profuse menstruation, as an aid to childbirth, and as a peerless nosebleed cure. It has been said that one whiff of the freshly-exposed root of the Trillium was sometimes enough to immediately halt the flow of blood. The leaves, though seldom taken internally, were boiled and mixed with lard to make a poultice for skin problems such as boils, sores, rashes, and ulcers. Since, according to their own testimony, Trillium was good for "any kind of sick," it's altogether possible that the the Yukis and the Wailakis used the plant for all these purposes too.

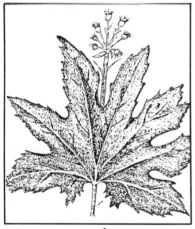

Western Coltsfoot

WESTERN COLTSFOOT

Petasites palmata

Other names for the Western Coltsfoot: This plant is also commonly known as Sweet Coltsfoot and Butter Bur. The Concow Indians used to call it *Ta-ta-te* and *Mal-e-me*. To the Wailaki it was *Tel-dink-to*, and to the Yuki, *Mul-com*.

Where to find it: The Coltsfoot is found on damp, shaded ground in many California locations. It is common especially along rivers and large streams in damp woodlands and in shady wooded places below 1,000 feet.

How to know it when you see it: On a single fat stem which boasts many coarse-looking leaf-like bracts arranged like scales, this robust, early-blooming perennial herb bears—like the head of a club—a terminal cluster of white or pinkish-white, sweet-scented flowers.

Its lore. Valued by some northern tribes for the salt that was easily obtained from the ashes of its green stems and leaves—a substance otherwise lacking in their largely-vegetarian diets—Western Coltsfoot was also prized for the medicinal properties of its rootstocks. From this underground rhizome the Concow, who called the root *Pe-we*, devised a medicine for treating the early stages of consumption. Sometimes too, the root was dried, pulverized, and applied in powder form as a treatment for boils and sores. Interestingly enough, the latter usage was a popular one for *Petasites* root elsewhere in the world, and notably, by people other than American Indians; the Elizabethan herbalist John Gerard suggested just such a treatment for sixteenth-century Englishmen. Sweet Coltsfoot has traditionally been used also as a remedy for intestinal worms, as a diuretic and an antispasmodic, and as a treatment for kidney stones.

Comment: Scientific tests conducted on animals indicate this plant may be cancer-causing if taken frequently or in large doses.

WILD GINGER

Asarum spp.

Other names for Wild Ginger: This plant is also known as Snakeroot, Colicroot, and Indian Ginger.

Where to find it: This member of the Birthwort family is found growing in cool woodlands and other wet and shady places where the soil is rich, especially in northern California. One species, *A. caudatum*, prefers deep shade in the coast range woods. Another, *A. lemmonii*, is found especially in Plumas and Sierra counties, while *A. hartwegi* prefers shaded places in Yellow Pine and Red Fir forests, at altitudes between 2,500 and 7,000 feet.

How to know it when you see it: Sometimes twining shrubs, sometimes low herbs, the Wild Ginger plants are best known for their lovely dark-green and heart-shaped leaves, their hairy stalks, and the triangular-tipped or slender-tailed, petal-like sepals of their often-drooping, brownish-red flowers. Like love notes tucked in folded paper valentines, these inconspicuous blooms are sometimes hidden beneath the leafy hearts.

Its lore. When V. K. Chestnut ran his studies on the ethnobiology of certain northern California tribes at the tail end of the nineteenth century and the beginning of the twentieth, he could find no record of their medicinal use of Wild Ginger, and yet, as he perceived it, the plant was so "remarkably aromatic" (unlike its own surprisingly foul-smelling flowers) that he couldn't help conjecturing that it must have been used at one time or other by the native medicine men. He may well have figured rightly. This much is certain: as a genus, all species of *Asarum* (Wild Ginger), fall under the classification, *Aristolochiaceae*, and are related, therefore, to the "Indian Root," which, according to Jose Longinos Martinez, who studied the flora of early California in 1792, was a very popular medicinal herb of California used as a powerful treatment for wounds and "ulcers in all stages." It's conceivable that in Martinez' day, California's Wild Ginger plants were used in much the same way and that they had simply fallen into disuse by the time Chestnut conjectured about it.

It's a known fact that Wild Ginger was considered a medicinal plant by Indians elsewhere in North America, as well as by settlers who chose to follow their ways. It was variously used as a remedy for heart palpitations, a medicament to normalize the menstrual cycle, a cure for intestinal gas and stomach cramps, and a tonic and appetite stimulant.

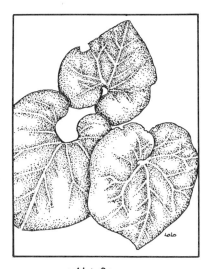

Wild Ginger

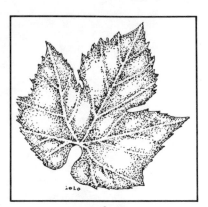

Wild Grape

WILD GRAPE

Vitis spp.

Other names for the Wild Grape: Other common English names for this plant are California Grape and Indian Grape. This was the beloved *Kop* of the Numlaki Indians, the *She-in* of the Pomo, the *Mot-mo mam* of the Yuki. The Cahuilla name for the plant was *Sawanawet*.

Where to find it: Not nearly so common as it was in California's halcyon days, when it seemed almost ubiquitous, the Wild Grape is still often found growing profusely along the banks of streams, in riverlands, and on slopes and foothills in various California locations.

How to know it when you see it: Similar to its cultivated kin, the Wild Grape is easily identified. Its vines are stout, its bark is shreddy, and its leaves—sometimes three-lobed, sometimes not—are broad and green.

Its lore. Most of the early visitors to California before the coming of the twentieth century had something to say, and to pen, about its superabundancy of lovely wild grapes. Among these were men like the observant young fortyniner, Peter Decker, who made note of the land's "pretty fine Grapes" in his famous diary, and the able journalist Edwin Bryant, who succumbed to a bit of purple prose when he described how the banks of the Sacramento River were fringed with Grape Vines, and what a charming sight it was. And consider the words of John Woodhouse Audubon, who visited California in the mid-nineteenth century. "At sundown, far down the valley of Santa Maria, we rejoined our camp and found all well, and Mr. Browning treated me to a pound or two of most delicious grapes. They tasted so refreshing and delicious, that for a few minutes I forgot everything else, all my anxieties for the termination of our long and tedious journey, with the attendant troubles and difficulties seemed smoothed over." Apparently there was no plant more representative of this far western land.

The California Indians seem to have used the Wild Grape frequently as a food, rarely as a medicinal. The northern Indians, who shared their habitat with *Vitis californica*, were quick to learn jelly-making from their settler neighbors, whom they helped in turn by teaching them where to find the tastiest and least sour fruit. (According to Yokia lore, the vines that festooned the Willow and Laurel trees produced tart fruit, while those that twined 'round the White and Black Oaks were sweeter, much better either fresh from the vine or preserved in luscious jellies and jams.) The Desert Indians not only ate the fruit of *V. girdiana* fresh from the vine, but added grapes to their stews, dried them as raisins, and, come the late nineteenth century, made them into a flavorful Wild Grape wine.

Perhaps the most interesting usage of the Wild Grape plant, and one that could be considered medicinal in a sense, was that of its vines at the hands of the Yurok Indians. Upon the death of a tribesman, anyone who had touched a corpse was believed to be dangerously contaminated and had to cleanse himself ceremoniously before he was safe. Ironically, this purification was effected by rubbing the body of the contaminated person with the very grapevine with which the corpse had been lowered into its grave.

It was the early settlers, however, who found the most medicinal uses for the various Wild Grapes that were ready for picking. They used concoctions made from the fruit as a tonic, a first-class "blood invigorator," a remedy for urinary problems, kidney stones, and bladder complaints, and as an eye wash. The leaves served to make poultices for cuts, scratches, sores, and snakebite.

WILD ONION

Allium spp.

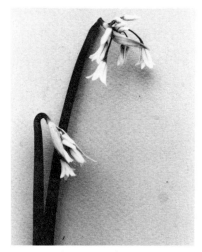

Nodding Onion

Other names for the Wild Onion: Species of this genus are variously known as Indian Onion, Nodding Onion, and Nodding Wild Onion. The Pomo Indian name for the Wild Onion was *Ko-bi-ye*. To the Yuki it was *Shep*; the Cahuilla name for *A. validum*, one of the Wild Onions that shared their habitat, was *Tep-ish*. The Spanish name for onion is *Cebolla*.

Where to find it: One species or another of this genus is found growing in almost every kind of habitat throughout the state. *A. unifolium*, a Wild Onion prized by several northern tribes, is found in moist and heavy soil at altitudes below 3,500 feet. *A. validum*, a particularly flavorful species and one well known to the desert Indians, favors altitudes that range from 4,000 to 11,000 feet. Another species, *A. biceptrum*, is at home in damp meadows, in Aspen groves and on moist banks up to 9,500 feet.

How to know it when you see it: Most of California's Wild Onions strongly resemble their cultivated kin. They are herbaceous plants boasting slim basal leaves and a showy head of flowers borne on the end of a stalk that, like the onion bulb itself, bears a distinctive and unmistakable oniony odor.

Its lore. Desert Indians like the Cahuilla looked upon the Wild Onion as a specific for stimulating the appetite and therefore, good medicine for the weak, the wan, and the convalescing. To many early settlers, however, this odiferous herb was probably much more than a simple tonic for the mildly ailing. This was especially likely with those who'd been schooled by the herbalists of the day, for many nineteenth-century experts were still under the influence of the famous plant wizard, Nicolas Culpeper, who'd once made far-reaching claims for the genus *Allium*. According to him, the common garden Onion could increase the sperm count in males, kill intestinal worms in children, cure headaches, soothe scalds and burns, and remove blemishes from the skin. The settlers may have doubted its efficacy on some of these counts, but they still believed that the onion (from the garden or from the wilds) could cure colds, ease hoarseness, relieve Poison Oak, and lessen the symptoms of asthma, rheumatism, and bronchitis.

The Onion has never fallen far from favor. Today some homoeopaths prescribe pills made from *Allium* (most often the garden variety) for the treatment of rhinitis and hay fever; many herbalists suggest an Onion-and-honey syrup as a remedy for coughs; and some wild-herb enthusiasts are beginning to experiment with Wild Onion poultices.

Warning: Experts warn that anyone in California who wishes to eat any of the Wild Onions should do so with caution. Never consume any part of a plant that looks like an Onion but does not have a strong Onion odor. True Onions always smell like Onions; this is the major key to their identity. Some plants that bear a strong resemblance to Onions, but do not have the familiar strong Onion scent, are not Onions at all but imposters so poisonous they can kill.

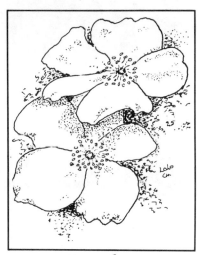

Wild Rose

WILD ROSE

Rosa spp.

Other names for the Wild Rose: Other English names for this lovely plant are Common Wild Rose, California Wild Rose, Wood Rose, Sweetbrier, and Brier Hip. The Cahuilla used to call it *Ushal*, while to the Yuki it was *Kal-e*. The Spanish name for the rose is *Rosa*.

Where to find it: Wild Roses are most often found in shaded and moist habitats at altitudes below 6,000 feet: places like the Truckee River country where Edwin Bryant delighted in the sight of them in 1846.

How to know it when you see it: California's Wild Roses are erect, sprawling, or climbing shrubs, covered with prickles, bearing alternate leaves in leaflets that number from five to seven, and flowers that boast a single row of five petals. These blooms, usually pinkish, evolve into plump red-to-orange seedpods that measure up to an inch in diameter and are commonly known as haws or hips. Since there are so many species of Wild Rose growing in the state of California and so much variation within a species, a detailed overall description is virtually impossible. Still, most roses are unmistakably roses; most are thorny and hard to handle; some bear a scent that's almost ethereal; all are medicinal and edible and lovely to see.

Its lore. No one needs to be told that the Rose is the most beloved of all flowers in the world. Roses are as beloved in California as in Massachusetts, as dear to the white man as to the Indian, as esteemed now as in the days when the native Americans were the only ones here to see them, to touch, pick, and eat them, or use them as medicine.

There's probably no plant in the world more capable of evoking romantic responses in those who come upon it suddenly in some unexpected setting, as Bryant did nearly a century and a half ago. As he perceived it, "the fragrant odor of the wild rose," coupled with the incense of the forest, was so evocative that it "melted the sensibilities, blunted as they were by long exposure and privation, and brought back to our memories the endearments of home and the pleasures of civilization."

Some northern California tribes, like the Yuki, only rarely used the Rose as food or medicine, however. And yet they esteemed it enough to give it a name—always a sure sign of a plant's importance. They must have valued their *Kal-e* largely for its beauty, then, or for the joy it was to catch a waft of its scent in the morning air. It was probably much the same with some of the southern tribes, like the Cahuilla, who occasionally found it growing in the swamps and along the washes and streams. Although it was at least a minor source of food for them, and they did make a pleasant-tasting beverage from its blossoms, it wasn't a common plant in their habitat, never a staple, never a major food or a stand-by medicine. Yet they too revered it enough to give it a name. It was *Ushal*, a sibilant word that seems somehow poignantly fitting since it can scarcely be mouthed without something akin to a sigh.

Early settlers too, delighted as they were to find this familiar beauty growing so abundantly in California, always looked to the Wild Rose primarily for its loveliness and only secondarily as a medicine. This was true in spite of the fact that the plant's medicinal uses were as familiar to them as those of Lydia Pinkham's bottled remedy on the counters back home. For centuries the Rose has been used as a treatment for bowel irregularity, colds, coughs, menstrual complications, and other common maladies.

Today some of California's herbalists use a rose-water preparation, derived from the Damask Rose, *Rosa Damascena*, as a soothing lotion for the eyes.

WILD RHUBARB

Rumex hymenosepalus

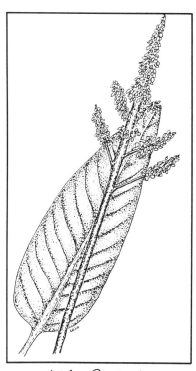

Wild Rhubarb

Other names for the Wild Rhubarb plant: Wild Rhubarb is also popularly known as Canaigre, Pie Plant, and Red Dock. The Cahuilla called this herb *Maalval*.

Where to find it: One of approximately twenty-four species of *Rumex* in California, Wild Rhubarb is a common perennial weed found in dry, sandy locations, in grasslands, coastal sage scrub, Joshua Tree woods, and Creosote Bush country, at altitudes mostly below 5,000 feet.

How to know it when you see it: The mostly-basal leaves of this plant, which is sometimes used as a substitute for Rhubarb, are smooth, fleshy, lance-shaped, and large. Measuring from six to eighteen inches in length, they're slightly wavy-edged and marked by a central vein. In spring, the upper halves of the stems bear small, rather unprepossessing green flowers, which mature into a cluster of much more conspicuous pinkish seedpods. A taste test helps to identify this species. Its leaves are extremely sour.

Its lore. To the southern Indians who may or may not have used this herb medicinally, Wild Rhubarb was valued especially for its roots, so rich in tannic acid, which served as a tanning agent in the preparation of hides. Other Californians, especially Hispanics, have used these same roots to make an externally-applied medicament for cuts and abrasions, or a mouthwash or gargle for minor oral complaints.

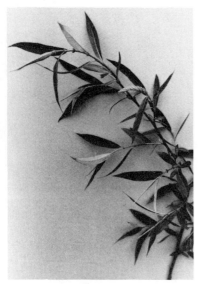

Willow

WILLOW

Salix lasiolepis and others

Other names for the Willow: Names for the various species of Willows found in California are Arroyo Willow, Pacific Willow, Red Willow, Mackenzie Willow, Black Willow, and others. To the Mojave Indians, the Willow was *Ihore*. The Pomo called one species, the Arroyo Willow, *Be-he*. To the Yokia this same tree was *Shka*. The Cahuilla name for the Black Willow was *Avasily*. *Ke-cham-ka* was the Cahuilla name given to a Willow identified by one writer as *S. Washingtonia*, a species which is not mentioned in authoritative works.

Where to find it: Since they root easily, Willows are sometimes found growing in dense thickets. Generally speaking, they're most at home along streams or other places where the soil is moist. The Arroyo Willow is common on stream banks and beds at altitudes lower than 7,000 feet in various California locations. Pacific Willow, another stream bank dweller, found at altitudes below 8,000 feet, grows all over the state except the desert. The Red Willow thrives in similar habitats, but is rarely found above 5,000 feet. The Mackenzie Willow, less common and more limited in its range than many of its relatives, is found in Red Fir forests at altitudes below 7,000 feet.

How to know it when you see it: Willows are deciduous shrubs or trees with light, soft wood that is generally pale, and alternate leaves that are usually much longer than they are broad. They bloom early in spring, sometimes before they're leaved, their tiny flowers attached to nectar-producing, hairy bracts. The fruit is a small capsule with two valves that are filled with many hairy seeds. Their winter buds are one of their most distinguishing features. Covered by a single scale, they hug the stems like animate creatures afraid of falling.

Its lore. The Willow is a lovely tree and does much to add to the ambience anywhere it grows. Edwin Bryant's description of those that he saw (in the company of Elms) near the Mission Santa Clara in the 1840s is well worth recording. It not only adds to the lore of the tree itself, but affords a charming glimpse into California's picturesque past.

"A broad alameda," Bryant wrote, "shaded by stately trees (elms and willows), planted by the padres, extends nearly the entire distance, forming a most beautiful drive or walk for equestrians or pedestrians. The motive of the padres in planting this avenue, was to afford the devout senoras and senoritas a shade from the sun, when walking from the Pueblo to the church at the mission to attend Mass."

That same species that afforded such welcome shade to the senoras and senoritas of old Santa Clara had already been serving the California Indians that purpose and many others for countless centuries. The Willow was unquestionably one of the Indian's most useful multipurpose plants. It was a substitute for chewing tobacco; dried and powdered, it served as mortar; it was the source of construction material for dozens of useful everyday items such as fish traps and tule-boats. It was a major medicinal plant too, its bark believed more beneficial than that of any other tree or shrub that grew in all the land, and the leaves themselves the source of many a worthwhile remedy. In this latter role it was widely used, greatly prized and, incidentally, never debunked. As a bark wash it was a treatment for itchy skin; as a leaf tea or a strong infusion it served as a peerless spring tonic. It cured chills, fever, and diarrhea when taken internally, or reduced the inflammation of sore eyes when used as eye-drops; it reduced the pains of arthritis, rheumatism, or the common headache. The ashes of burned twigs were mixed with water and employed to treat venereal diseases. Dried and powdered root was applied to the navels of newborn babies and sprinkled over hard-to-heal sores of every variety. The bark and seeds were stuffed up the nostrils to stop nose bleeds, and placed in the mouth to ease the pain of a toothache. Steeped in water or wine, the roots, bark, and leaves made a hair rinse good for dandruff control. And as the Mojaves well knew, a wad of Willow leaves, held in the mouth like chewing tobacco, helped foot-weary travelers ward off thirst.

Many of these same uses were known to the settlers, to whom Willow cures were never a surprise. Words of the wonders wrought by this tree had been on the lips of their grandparents and on the pages of their herbals for as long as they could remember.

Since it's common knowledge today that the Willow contains salicin, and that this is the substance from which aspirin is derived, no one questions the fact that this tree was beneficial to the old-timers who made medicinal use of it. Herbalists are still using its bark and leaves today, especially in the preparation of health-giving tonics not much different from those concocted a hundred years ago.

WOOD SORREL

Oxalis spp.

Other names for the Wood Sorrel: This woodland plant is also known as Shamrock, Sorrel, White Wood Sorrel, and Sour Trefoil.

Where to find it: Most species of this genus are at home in moist, shady soils, in woodlands, in rocky places, and on moss-covered banks. *Oxalis oregana*, for example, best known as Redwood Sorrel, is distinctly a shade plant and is found in Redwood and Douglas Fir forests from Monterey County upward. Suksdorf's Wood Sorrel favors damp shaded spots also in forests and woodlands. *Oxalis californica*, however, has other tastes entirely. It's common on dry, brushy slopes, in stony soil, in coastal sage scrub, and chaparral in more southerly parts of the state.

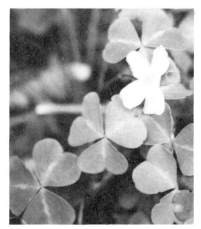

Wood Sorrel

How to know it when you see it: The typical Wood Sorrel is a perennial woodsdweller, low to the ground, cool to the touch, fast-spreading on its creeping rootstock. It's a charming plant with Clover-like leaves that are a true green on top, purplish on their undersides. Each leaf is comprised of three heart-shaped leaflets, which are joined at their tips and borne by slender round stems that range in color from pale green to reddish. The delicately-veined flowers are five-petaled, and usually rise up a little higher than the leaves that surround them as if arranged by someone who wanted to make sure they weren't missed. The flowers of Creeping Wood Sorrel and several other species are yellow, while those of the Redwood Sorrel are white or pinkish. The plants are sour to the taste.

Its lore. When they first set foot in California, the settlers must have delighted in finding that Wood Sorrel, which they'd prized in their gardens in the east, was thriving in the woodlands of this vibrant new land. Although there are no records to show that they did, it's probable that they began to use the plant here much as they had back home: as the source of a very fine tea, said to be good for quenching thirst, strengthening a weak stomach, or combating kidney problems.

Today some herbalists still suggest the use of Wood Sorrel preparations, especially as a wash or lotion for dry or chapped skin, rashes, or sunburn.

Warning: The leaves of Wood Sorrel contain oxalic acid, which may cause diarrhea, kidney stones, kidney failure, or hemorrhaging if taken internally in large amounts.

Excessive consumption over an extended period of time may inhibit the absorption of calcium by the body.

WORMWOOD

Artemesia spp.

Other names for Wormwood: Other common English names for Wormwood are Mugwort, Madderwort, and Sagebrush. The Pomo Indian name for one species (the well known Mugwort, *A. Douglasiana*), was *Komp-lu-li*. To the Yokia this same herb was *Ka-blu*. To the Cahuilla, California Sagebrush (*A. californica*) was *Hulvel*; Basin Sagebrush (*A. trindentata*) was *Wikwat*. Three popular Spanish names for Wormwood are *Altamisa, Alcachfa,* and *Arcacil*.

Where to find it: One well known Wormwood, the one most often referred to as Mugwort, is found growing in waste places, arroyos, canyons, and fields at altitudes below 6,000 feet, in various California locations. California Sagebrush favors dry slopes and fans at altitudes below 2,500 feet. Basin Sagebrush is most apt to be found on slopes and dry plains, in woodlands, and on the edges of deserts at far ranging altitudes of between 1,500 and 10,600 feet. *A. ludoviciana*, another species often used medicinally, leans toward dry, open places at altitudes below 8,500 feet.

How to know it when you see it: With all the medicinal Wormwood plants, odor is as telltale a feature as appearance. These herbs or shrubs, which vary so greatly in size and shape, are always aromatic, distinctly pungent, and unquestionably "medicine-y." Their smell is one that's best described as a cross between Sage and Camphor. Another distinguishing feature is the hairiness of the leaves, which tend to bear a grayish cast. These leaves are occasionally lance-shaped, more often deeply cleft, but sometimes rather like unkempt flannel fringe or the whangs on an old buckskin garment long overdue for the trash heap. The flowers of the Wormwoods are small roundish balls borne along the stem in unleafed rows that are generally one-sided.

Its lore. To the Ohlone Indians, whose tule-boats once left their ruffling wakes in the San Francisco Bay, Wormwood (probably the variety known as Mugwort) was more than a remedy, it was a charm against ills and misfortunes of every variety, a protection for both the body and the mind. Sprigs of the plant served as a kind of good luck talisman—worn about the neck in the same manner as latter-day Spaniards were to wear their holy medals—to ward away thoughts and dreams and harmful reveries about the dead.

Hundreds of miles away, in southern California, the Cahuilla Indians, especially the women of the tribe, regarded another *Artemisia*, the California Sagebrush, in much the same way. A tea brewed from this herb was a ceremonial drink as well as a medicine, a potion that prepared young girls for womanhood, strengthened them and kept them pure and clean, helped them to maintain their monthly fast, and literally assisted them through every step of their life thereafter. It saved them from menstrual pains and distress; it helped them ease their way through menopause; it was a comfort on the day of childbirth. Even newborn babies were given this drink to flush out their systems.

Leaves of the same plant, like those of the Basin Sagebrush, were used by women and men alike as a remedy for common colds, and as a sweathouse inhalant good for all sorts of ailments, especially rheumatic aches and pains. In like manner the Yuki of Round Valley used the Mugwort, and likewise the settlers who came to share their habitat.

Because of their past experience with Wormwood, newcomers to California were probably predisposed to accept all of the *Artemisia* plants that they found growing in the land. It was no wonder that they were. In the old world, Mugwort had been used as a "childbirth herb," as a treatment for palsy and epilepsy, and as a traveler's remedy, a charm to protect wayfarers from ailments that ran the gamut from general weariness to sore feet.

Even today Wormwood is sometimes used as a foot soak, a sauna bath, a stomach tonic, and, as the Cahuilla women might have foreseen, as a soothing tea for easing the pains of menstrual cramps.

The leaves of this herb have recognized value as an insect repellent—a virtue that was much to the advantage of early settlers who used to sprinkle the dried leaves into their bedrolls to ward away fleas.

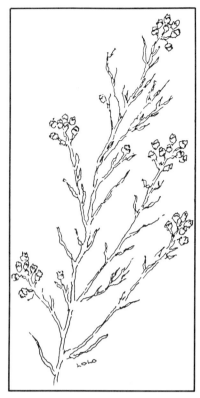

Wormwood

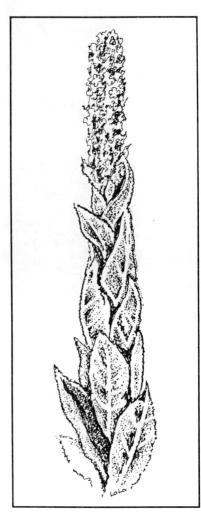

Woolly Mullein

WOOLLY MULLEIN

Verbascum thapsus

Other names for Woolly Mullein: This plant is also known as Common Mullein, Velvet Plant, Candlewick, Blanket Leaf, Aaron's Rod, Mullein Dock, Flannel Mullein, Flannel-leaf, Old Man's Flannel, Feltwort, Hare's Beard, Peter's Staff, Juniper's Staff, Shepherd's Club, and Hedge Taper. The Spanish name for Woolly Mullein is *Gordolobo*.

Where to find it: At home in waste places, such as river bottoms and ditches, this alien from Eurasia is a common weed in California, especially in the northern part of the state. It's most at home at altitudes above 4,000 feet, yet is often found in lower places too, as in Sonoma and Mendocino counties where it can be seen growing by the sides of roads, in ditches and gullies, and on vacant land.

How to know it when you see it: Just think about the various monikers by which this plant is known and you'll find it easy enough to identify. Its great basal leaves, which form a neat grayish rosette, are as velvety as a dog's ear. The stout stalk that rises up from this cushiony base (covered with tight buds, modest yellow flowers, seed pods and yet more up-pointing velvety leaves) calls to mind unquestionably a staff, a rod, a walking stick. Touch the plant. Finger its leaves with your eyes closed and you might as well have your hands on some scraps of good thick flannel.

Its lore. Apparently the Woolly Mullein was not one of those introduced plants that the Indians took to heart at once and began to use medicinally. Some tribesmen did occasionally add its leaves to the tobacco they smoked in their pipes, but other than that it seems to have found no place in their lives or their folk medical lore. It did have a place in the lore of other Californians, however, for among English-speaking peoples it was a plant with a long and colorful history of medicinal use. Herbalists in England and America alike touted a Mullein flower oil as a remedy for piles and a Mullein leaf decoction as a cure for cramps, convulsions, coughs and toothaches. Some modern herbalists still praise the plant today and suggest its use as a mild sedative for the lungs, good for easing coughs and chest infections.

YARROW

Achillea spp.

Other names for Yarrow: More common English names for this plant are Milfoil, Old Man's Pepper, Thousand-leaved, Nosebleed, Thousand-seal, Dog Daisy, Knight's Milfoil, and Soldier's Woundwort. To the Yuki Indians it was *Nun-alt-mil*. A Spanish name for Yarrow is *Plumajillo*.

Where to find it: This perennial from Eurasia, naturalized in the east probably long before it reached the far west, is found in lawns, in old fields, at the edges of woodlands, by paths and roads, and in open clearings in various California locations.

How to know it when you see it: Each slender, linear leaf of this aromatic plant is like a work of art designed by an engraver or a scrimshander or some other master craftsman with a keen eye for detail. Its every dissected leaflet is like a duplicate of itself, equally lacy, equally intricate, just as much a work of art. Yarrow blossoms (actually many little heads of flowers with only a few flowers per head) are usually white, sometimes pinkish, and are congregated together in flat pie-like clusters that form in different places along the stem.

Its lore. A tea made from the Yarrow plant was highly prized by some of the northern Indians as a treatment for such diverse ailments as headaches and consumption, while an extract of the plant served as a liniment for bruises and sprains. Desert Indians used the same herb as a mouthwash for toothache and pyorrhea. Significantly enough, settlers had many similar uses for this versatile old-timer, as had their parents and their grandparents before them. This was the same plant that the Old World herbalists had esteemed ever since the dauntless Achilles, hero of Homer's Iliad, administered it to his soldiers to stanch the blood of their battle wounds. This was always its greatest claim to glory—its legendary ability to halt a flow of blood—whether from battle wound or nosebleed, dog bite or bleeding gums. But its uses were never limited; it was employed to treat a never-ending list of common maladies, ills that ranged from earaches to piles.

   Used most often in the form of a tea or a poultice and believed to be anti-inflammatory and astringent, Yarrow is still a much-respected herb today.

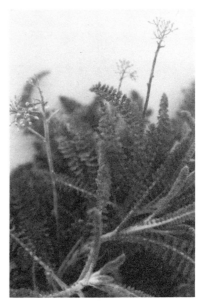

Yarrow

YERBA BUENA

Satureja douglasii

Other names for Yerba Buena: The popular name of this plant was bequeathed it by the Spaniards. Literally, it means "Good Herb." The Luiseno Indians used to call it *Huvamel.* To the Concow it was *Bul-luk-to,* to the Yokia *Ma-stit.*

Where to find it: This little native vine which once grew so abundantly on the soil where the city of San Francisco stands today, is a moisture-loving plant, happiest in shady spots, in coastal scrub, in Redwood forests, in chaparral, mixed evergreen woodlands, and in shaded ravines in many California locations. It seems to favor especially the lovely Point Reyes Peninsula, where it keeps company with plants such as the shiny-leaved Salal, Cow Parsnip, Pearly Everlasting, a few wild grasses, and an assortment of ferns.

How to know it when you see it: Like other mints, Yerba Buena boasts square stems, opposite leaves, and a pleasing aroma. In other ways it seems to part

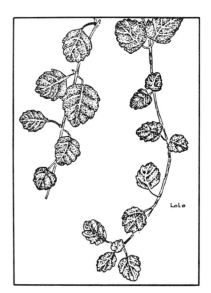

Yerba Buena

company with its kin. It's a dainty, trailing vine instead of an upright plant like Horehound and many other mints. Its round to ovate leaves, which have a vague sheen like a fine patina, lack the crinkly look typical to those of many other mints, and appear much smoother, although they're slightly sandpapery to the touch.

Its lore. Early Spaniards in California—Californios, as they called themselves—came to love this little trailing vine that they found growing so profusely in the vast new land. They prized it so highly, in fact, that it inspired the first name they ever attached to the settlement that later grew up to be San Francisco. Yerba Buena, they called it in its early days. And in that era they used the aromatic mint in question as the makings of a fine beverage that was not only refreshing and good tasting, but marvelously medicinal. Just as the Indians did, they used this tea as a tonic to purify the blood, to aid digestion, to relieve colic, to induce restful sleep, and to lessen the pains of arthritis. Perhaps they even followed the practice of the Cahuilla and the Luiseno and bound the vines around their heads to cure their headaches.

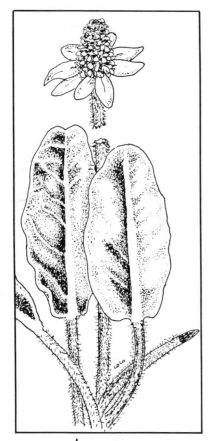

Yerba Mansa

YERBA MANSA

Anemopsis californica

Other names for Yerba Mansa: Another common English name for this plant is Lizard Tail. To the Cahuilla Indians it was *Chivnish*.

Where to find it: Yerba Mansa is a common plant in lowland meadows and in wet, alkaline places below 6,500 feet, in the Sacramento Valley, in Santa Clara and Inyo counties, and in many southern California locations.

How to know it when you see it: Yerba Mansa is a highly specialized and very unusual-looking plant. Once seen, it's immediately recognized forever thereafter. One-half to two feet tall, it bears a cluster of many flowers, encircled by white bracts, which are so deceptively petal-like that the overall impression is that of one flower only: a single, beautiful, star-like bloom with a cone in its center, bound to catch the eye of any passerby. The true flowers, which are encircled by those prestidigitating bracts, are quite minute and bear no petals whatsoever. The stem-clasping leaf blades of the plant are oblong to oval.

Its lore. Like Yerba Buena and Yerba Santa, this plant was an old Indian herb of considerable repute that was quickly adopted by the early Spanish population. And so valued was this wondrous plant that the Californios who lived outside the range of its habitat, such as those who dwelt in Yerba Buena country, would go to great lengths to acquire it, even if it meant that they had to travel miles on horseback or pay large sums to those who did. Once the herb was in their hands, they put it to use after the fashion of the Indians from whom they'd learned of its prowess. They peeled, mashed, squeezed, and boiled its aromatic roots and then drank the resulting decoction to treat cases of pleurisy, ulcers, colds, indigestion, asthma, and chest congestion. They chopped up the bark and used it to make a brew that served as a wash, a lotion, or a liniment for aches, pains, and stubborn sores. They made poultices from crushed leaves and used these to relieve rheumatism and reduce swelling. They cut, dried, and pulverized all parts of the plant and sprinkled this precious powder over knife wounds and other lacerations to disinfect them and insure their speedy healing. With all of these preparations they also treated their horses, dogs, and other animals just as the Indians had done for so many years.

Yerba Mansa was a true cure-all, a much-respected herb that was widely used by Hispanic Californians well into this century, and is still a trusted remedy for a few loyal users.

YERBA SANTA

Eriodictyon californicum and *E. trichocalyx*

Other names for Yerba Santa: Translated from the Spanish, the most popular name for this old medicinal herb, "Yerba Santa," means nothing less than "holy herb." The plant is also sometimes known as Mountain Balm, Wild Balsam, or Gum Leaves. To the Little Lake Indians it was *Sa-tek*; to the Concow, *Wa-sa-got-o*; to the Yuki, *Til-at-mil*; to the Cahuilla *Tanwivel*.

Where to find it: One species of this plant, *E. californicum*, is found on dry ridges, rocky slopes, and brushy hillsides, in chaparral, and in Pine and mixed evergreen and Redwood forests at altitudes below 5,500 feet, especially in the northern part of the state. Another species, *E. trichocalyx*, which can be found at altitudes up to 8,000 feet, also favors dry places such as rocky slopes and fans, but finds these spots in southern California's Joshua Tree and Pinyon-Juniper woods instead of the tall Pine and Redwood forests of the north.

How to know it when you see it: Five to seven feet high, the "holy herb" is an aromatic, resinous, evergreen shrub with shreddy bark, alternate leaves that are leathery and irregularly toothed, and many white to purplish flowers that are borne in flat-topped clumps or clusters.

Leaves of this plant tend to blacken with age, the result of a fungus that overtakes them.

Its lore. This herb, the "holy herb," extolled by the mission padres and their flocks, was important to Indian tribes all over the land. Here was the *Til-at-mil* of the Yuki, the *Sa-tek* of the Little Lake, the *Wa-sa-got-o* of the Concow: a cure for grippe, rheumatism, consumption, catarrh, colds, and asthma. Here was the much-esteemed *Tanwivel* of the Desert Indians in the south, who used it for the same purposes the northerners did, and a couple more in addition. They

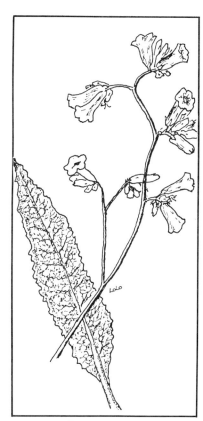

Yerba Santa

bound its fresh pounded leaves to fatigued and aching limbs; they chewed those leaves to quench their thirst when water was nowhere in sight.

How many of these uses were employed by the Spaniards, and by the other settlers who came trekking into California, no one really knows. But that new-comers used this herb medicinally and prized it greatly is a well-known fact. They found it to be the source of a very refreshing beverage too, one that they sometimes mixed with Horehound, sometimes with whiskey, and sometimes used to disguise the taste of Quinine, one of the few other medicines they needed when they had a quantity of this holiest of holy herbs on hand.

3
Origins of Diseases According to Early Californians. Who Got Sick? Who Died? And Why?

Blindness of an Indian woman. According to beliefs shared by many tribes of California Indians, the victim may havc engaged in basket weaving when she was menstruating, at which time such employment was strictly forbidden.

Boils suffered by forty-niners. In the days of the goldrush, boils were believed to have been caused by bruises contracted while mining.

Chills and fever in miners. These symptoms were thought to be caused by spending the night in some dank lowland spot by the side of a river.

Childbirth, difficult. If a Yurok woman suffered much pain when her child was born, both she and her tribefolk immediately suspected that she had slept too much while she was pregnant.

Drowsiness and enfeeblement of a Mojave Indian fisherman. In keeping with an old Mojave legend, the weakened Indian may have eaten fish that were caught in his net while that contrivance was still brand new. The ghosts of the fish, the *Nyavedhi*, may have taken away his shadow, his *Matkwesa*. If this were the case, he could not gain back his soul without the aid of a shaman, whose song could make him well again.

Granulated eyelids of a Luiseno woman. Consistent with tribal beliefs, the maiden may have consumed a portion of venison or jack rabbit during a prescribed period of abstinence.

Headaches. Concordant with the convictions of some coffee-loving California settlers, morning headaches often followed an evening supper at which no caffeine had been served. A copious quantity of coffee, of course, was the only known cure. In the nineteenth century, this much-favored beverage was considered highly medicinal.

Illness, otherwise inexplicable, of a Chukchansi Indian. In accordance with tribal beliefs, an ill-intentioned shaman may have blown tobacco smoke upon the victim. Depending on his or her inclinations, a Chukchansi medicine doctor could either cause a sickness or enact a cure by this same simple action.

Illness of settler women. They may have been riding about the country dressed in men's clothing, in which case—at least in the eyes of some menfolk—they were simply getting their just dues. According to forty-niner Peter Decker, women became ill ". . . from going about clad in men's clothes . . ." and from shamelessly traveling ". . . from town to town in this country on horseback." Decker was plainly scandalized. "Such is a specimen of California morals," he righteously declared.

Illness of a Yuki infant. The parents may have eaten salt or fat soon after the birth of their child, food strictly forbidden them during the first few days of the child's life.

Illness of a Yurok Indian. The victim may have drunk water from a stream that was contaminated by a drowned dog or by the presence of a *Sa'aitl*, a ghostly dwarf-like creature who barked like a dog and who frequently haunted overgrown creeks. Cases of illness in which contaminated water didn't seem to be the cause may have been attributable to *Ohpok* poisoning. *Ohpok* was the name of a deadly poison that was compounded of rattlesnake or frog, dog flesh, and salamander larva.

Hair loss of an Indian woman. Instead of using the prescribed scratching bone or scratching stick, she had scratched her head with her hand during her monthly period, when such behavior was strictly forbidden. This belief was shared by many California tribes.

Painful symptoms of a Wyot Indian. It was believed that self-moving, soft, transparent, worm-like objects had somehow invaded his or her body. These were the actual pains: tangible entities that could only be removed by the powers of a shaman.

Paralysis of a Huchnom Indian girl. She may have walked about in the sight of men during that time of the month when her presence was considered distinctly contaminating and the possible occasion of evil.

Pimples on the face of a Luiseno Indian girl. She must have scratched herself with her hand instead of with the stick prescribed for this purpose.

Sudden death of a Hupa Indian. A spiritually-delivered material object called a *Kitdonghoi*, usually a mysterious arrow, may have been shot at the victim, and a particular formula simultaneously incanted by an evil layperson (not a shaman) who was referred to in the same manner as the offending object: he or she was also a called a *Kitdonghoi*.

Sudden death of a Maidu Indian. Just one glimpse of the ghost of a deceased relative may have proved enough to kill a surviving Maidu.

Sudden death of a Pomo child. The shadow of a shaman's medicine bundle may have fallen across the path of the victim. The shamans' bags of treasures contained such items as bones, roots, dried lizards, coyote feet, and colored pebbles—fetishes so powerful that tender young humans could not withstand the force of a bundle's image if it were inadvertantly (or intentionally) cast upon them.

Sudden death of a Wintun Indian. The victim may have been struck by a particularly destructive *Dokos* (pain), delivered via the occult workings of an enemy. The word *Dokos* means an obsidian or flint arrow point, and is descriptive of the Wintun Indian perception of pain. To this tribe, as to many other native Californians, every ache or pain was perceived as a tangible object. In the case of the Wintun, it was a kind of occult arrow point, or in the words of the anthropologist A. L Kroeber, a "spirit missile."

Sudden death of a Yokut Shaman. The victim may have suffered the wages of a secret attack of a *Kuyohock*, a "shaman killer."

Swelling or choking of the internal organs of a Yurok Indian. This condition, called *Upunamitle*, was generally caused by witchcraft or by the breaking of an important taboo.

4
Old-Time California Remedies From House and Garden

ASAFETIDA

Narthex asafoetida and allied plants

Every band of settlers that made its way to California in the nineteenth century boasted at least a few avid Asafetida users in its ranks, individuals who were convinced that this smelly substance, aptly nicknamed "Devil's Dung" (really the resinous gum of an umbelliferous plant from central Asia), was not only a cure-all but a preventive medicament that could ward off ailments of every variety. It was sometimes worn about the neck like an amulet, a lucky charm so potent that it could hold even the devil at bay. As one California-bound forty-niner commented in his diary ". . . Dr. Boyle gave Asafetida as a preventative & it smells enough to keep off cholera & everybody else."

Asafetida was still in common use in California households well into the twentieth century. "My mother used to break a piece of Asafetida off and put it in a piece of cloth," says Dorothy L. Cooper, an herb-wise woman of Plantina, California. She goes on to explain how this "Asafetida treatment" was administered, a simple enough procedure, albeit odoriferous. All the Asafetida user need do was take that piece of cloth, ". . . tie it with a string and wear it around your neck all winter to keep away germs."

Another Californian, octogenarian Viola Vallier, who moved to Los Angeles from Illinois in the early 1920s, has keen recollections of Asafetida: "It was awful," she says, wrinkling her nose to accentuate her firm conviction. "I hated it. But my grandparents had drilled into my head how important it could be to a person's health. I felt guilty when I didn't hang it about the necks of my children."

BORAGE

Borago officinalis

This fine old classic herb, under cultivation in California as early as 1825 (when it was thriving in the gardens of Don Jose Maria de Estudillo, the one-time commandant of San Diego), is as beloved to humans as it is to bees. It's not a beauteous plant in itself, but it's fully redeemed by its remarkable flowers, black-anthered blue stars so unique, so lovely, they've inspired generations of avid needleworkers. They're depicted in so many motifs for embroidery designs they are literally a part of our country's folk art.

It's interesting to note that Borage was such a respected medicinal in the time of Estudillo that it was one of seven prized herbs the aristocratic old "Californio" packed and shipped to a friend in Hawaii in January of 1826—a return favor for some thread, a bit of sealing wax, and six bottles of something called Zumo de limon, which that friend, Don Francisco de Paula Marin, had shipped to *him* from Honolulu.

Of all the popular remedies of the day, none was more highly esteemed than *Borago officinalis*, which had as many claims to fame (whether warranted or not) as any modern miracle drug can boast today. Here was a prime ingredient of soothing teas and poultices. Here was a tonic to fortify the heart and strengthen the limbs. Here was a treatment for kidney ailments, bladder infection, pulmonary troubles, and assorted fevers. Here too was a laxative (mild but sure), an aid to digestion, a remedy for jaundice, a lotion for inflamed eyes, a ringworm cure, an herb to increase the milk supply in nursing mothers, and a supposed cure for the stings of insects and the bites of reptiles and rabid dogs.

Claims of Borage's wondrous healing powers neither began nor ended with the Spanish Dons. When American settlers began to trickle into this land of earthquakes and grizzly bears, they brought with them all their own remedies, amongst them—yes, of course—the selfsame Borage. This was no coincidence, for the fame of this old medicinal plant was age-old and worldwide.

CAMPHOR

Cinnamomum camphora

In the nineteenth century this crystalline substance from the wood of Formosa's medicinal Camphor tree too often proved dangerous in the hands of early settlers. It was a valuable medicament if used with care, of course. It served as a wonderful liniment for bruises, sprains, and aches, and a good rub for a congested chest. But when administered carelessly by uninformed men and women whose circumstances compelled that they doctor themselves, the results were sometimes calamitous. The journalist Edwin Bryant wrote poignantly of just such an occasion. A certain traveler, whose name he did not know, leaped from his wagon ". . . under the influence of a paroxysm of insanity with loud cries and shrieks . . ." It took two or three men to get the unfortunate fellow in tow. After several hours he began to appear less agitated, but by that time he was suffering from extreme nausea, yet unable to vomit until given an emetic. Ultimately, according to Bryant, ". . . he threw up nearly an ounce of the concrete gum of camphor." He'd taken the medication the day before to treat some pains that one can safely assume were minor compared to the woes induced by the medicine he took to treat them.

Well into the twentieth century, Californians, like other Americans, often resorted to potentially hazardous self-medication. Ironically, the books on their shelves, to which they turned to widen their knowledge, often bid them do just this. Mrs. Charles A. Reuter of Tehachapi, California still has in her possession one of her mother-in-law's favorites, a copy of the "White House Cook Book," published in 1905, which contains a recipe for removing tartar from the teeth—a formula that calls for one ounce of pure muriatic acid!

CHILI PEPPER

Capsicum frutescens

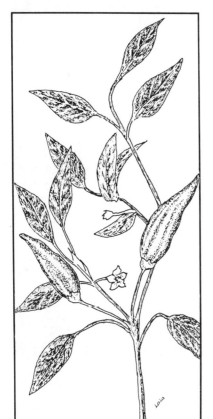

Chili Pepper

Despite Capsicum's long history as a medicinal herb, early Californians looked upon their beloved Chili Pepper more as a condiment than as a medicine. True, they realized that it was good for them; that the food to which it was added was both slow to spoil and easy to digest. They knew that a Chili Pepper liniment eased away the pains of rheumatism, arthritis, and bursitis. It was a perfectly good medicament—but this was not the prime reason for prizing it. They frankly loved its taste. It was a food one found everywhere in this far western land. Whether visiting in the rancho of Dona Maria Ygnacia Carrillo in Santa Rosa, or in the home of the noble centenarian, Senora Dona Guadalupe Briones de Miramontes of Spanishtown (Half Moon Bay), a sojourner in California could expect to dine on Chili Peppers at every meal—including breakfast.

In the first half of the nineteenth century, a typical California morning repast consisted of warm bread, frijoles, coffee, and stewed beef accompanied with, yes, the ever-ubiquitous, only-incidentally-medicinal Chili Pepper. Chili Pepper for breakfast, Chili Pepper for lunch, Chili Pepper for supper; this was the order of the day. In the words of one early resident, William Heath Davis, Jr., ". . . red peppers were their favorite seasoning." A newcomer himself, Hawaiian born—though schooled in the manners of his Bostonian forebears—and much more accustomed to bland foods than the tongue-scorching Capsicum, he couldn't help remarking that the Californios' "meat stews were excellent when not too highly seasoned with red pepper."

Even the gardens of the middle class Californios, which, unlike the grandiose horticultural displays on the grounds of the aristocracy, generally boasted little else than potatoes, onions, and frijoles (beans), were most conspicuous for their rows of showy red peppers. Except for the Indians' acorn mush and fine spring Clover, there was probably no food more representative of early California.

Some herbalists today are of the opinion that the legendary good health of the early Californio was at least partially attributable to their regular consumption of this old-fashioned favorite.

COFFEE

"Strong coffee quenches thirst best of anything (as men know who travel here)," averred forty-niner Peter Decker, who, along with many another gold-seeker, never tired of singing the praises of this standby beverage, which he viewed as a medicament almost as valuable as camphor or quinine. One day he ". . . met two Illiniois boys camped sick & without animals;" he passed ". . . Readings Bar which has yielded richly;" he spent midday on the river bank where he was feeling very ill. "Had fever," he explained, "my head seemed pierced by a thousand needles & my joints & back in particular ached to distress. Drank a pint of hot coffee, sweat profusely & got better."

COMFREY

Symphytum asperum

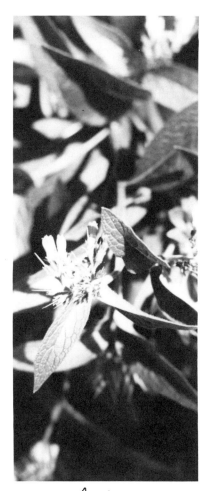

Comfrey

Of all the old American folk remedies, this alien from Asia may well be the most well known of all. This stands true in California as surely as it does elsewhere in the United States. Ask the man in the street to name a medicinal herb and chances are the word "Comfrey" will come to his lips.

In spite of all this, Comfrey's role in early California folk medicine is not a typical one. A late-comer, it never was a favorite with the Indians. And as for the Spaniards, apparently these well-versed herbalists preferred to cultivate its relative, Borage. It was the latter-day settlers, the Americans and Europeans, who really took this tough old foreigner to heart. And, since Comfrey's greatest claim to fame was its reputed powers to heal damaged bones and ligaments, it's no wonder that they did. In this new land where hazards were many, accidents were frequent, and doctors were few, it was exactly what they needed.

Comfrey was extolled as an effective treatment for a vast assortment of other conditions too, including rheumatism, arthritis, tuberculosis, asthma, and internal ulcers. Applied externally, in juice form or in a poultice made of either bruised leaves or mashed-root, it was an application to beautify the complexion, remove wrinkles, help heal sores, draw out festering splinters, hasten the healing of scratches and burns, soothe swollen breasts, and cure the infected navels of newborn babes. Taken internally, in the form of tea, it was a favorite general remedy of countless early settlers.

"In the old days," reflects Dorothy L. Cooper of Platina, California, "herbs were used by all oldtimers," and she goes on to explain quite plainly why this was so: "because most places a doctor was not available." It was as simple as that. Yet it's interesting to note that even today, when California physicians abound, Comfrey is still a favorite stand-by cure-all with many residents, Ms. Cooper included. "I heard Comfrey was poison," she says, "but it's the best herb when you aren't feeling well. I have used it for years. Tea of it makes you feel great."

Warning: Despite its lengthy history of safe consumption, recent discoveries show that continuous internal use of Comfrey may cause cancer.

CREAM OF TARTAR

A popular item in the settler's pantry, Cream of Tartar (purified and crystallized bitartrate of potassium) also had its place in many a nineteenth-century medicine chest, in the saddle bags of would-be doctors, in the wagon master's cure-all box, and in the battered valises of countless weary miners. Administered for a vast assortment of ailments, it was sometimes mixed with sulfur and given as a tonic and blood purifier.

DANDELION

Taxaxacum officinale

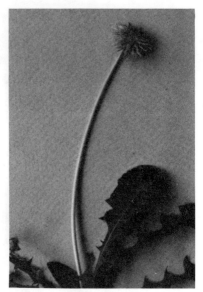

Dandelion

Dandelion ranks right along with Comfrey as a medicinal herb everyone seems to know. Dandelion tea, Dandelion wine, Dandelion tonic—all these preparations have a familiar ring. Whether one has tasted them or not seems almost irrelevant; the point is that everyone has heard of them. Like Paul Bunyan or Davy Crockett, they're a part of the lore of the land.

Early settlers used Dandelion, as it's still used by its enthusiasts today, for the treatment of a long list of physical complaints. As a tincture, fluid extract, or in powder form, it's a traditional home remedy for acne, boils, psoriasis, and various other skin ailments. As a tea or strong infusion, it has been used for indigestion, jaundice, diabetes, and low blood sugar. In decoctions it's a suggested medicament for anemia, bronchitis, constipation, gallstones, and kidney diseases. It is widely lauded as a bracing tonic, a soothing tea, a gentle laxative, an excellent restorative herb for individuals recovering from hepatitis, and as a superlative treatment for an assortment of digestive ailments.

KEROSENE (COAL OIL)

As a standby household remedy, an everyday cure-all for children, chickens, and dogs alike, there was a time in the late nineteenth and early twentieth centuries when this homely substance may have been the most commonly used of all. In the words of Platina's Dorothy L. Cooper, ". . . Kerosene was used to swab the throats of children three times a day for diptheria. Those who used it seemed to make it through."

MELONS

Along with Grapes, Blackberries, and Chili Pepper, melons bore mention in many descriptions of early California. It's true that their health-giving properties were not as widely sung as their taste. It's also true that, despite the fact that they're a natural diuretic, that they're enormously thirst quenching, that they could even save lives in times and places where available water is unsafe to drink, the melon never has ranked high on herbalists' lists of medicinal plants. Nonetheless, in the eighteenth and nineteenth centuries, most Europeans considered the seeds of this nutritious food, along with those of the Pumpkin, the Gourd and the Cucumber, as worthy of the place they filled in the medical pharmacopoeias of the day. Since California had its share of European immigrants (and of Americans whose folk medical practice they'd influenced), we can rest assured that the health-affording attributes of the melons of the land were not discounted. Certainly they must have been furthered by the high-quality specimens that were raised at the famous settler's way-station, Sutter's Fort, and at that establishment's agricultural showplace, the once-famous Hock Farm. The Captain's mistress, a Hawaiian woman by the name of Manaiki, whose life story is shrouded in mystery, was once known all over the Sacramento Valley, not only for her illicit affair with the Swiss gentleman who came to be known as "the father of California," but also for the wonderful melons she grew in her garden.

OLIVES

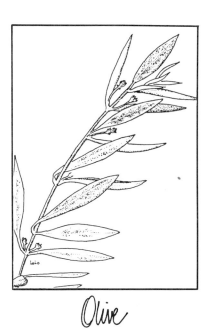

Olive

From the time the mission padres first introduced it in 1796, many early Californios took great pride in cultivating this lovely long-lived tree, the branch of which is a symbol of peace, the fruit of which yields the world's most famous cosmetic and medicinal oil. Among these gentlemen was the horticulturally-inclined Don Jose M. de Estudillo, who prided himself on his Olives. Once he magnanimously shipped starter slips of the tree to a friend across the sea, but not until after he'd done all he could to assure himself they'd not be neglected. In a letter, written well in advance of the shipment, he wrote: ". . . the olive trees will go to you also in a box with the slips placed in a planting crate. But I charge you at the same time, or any other friend who comes to the coast to receive it, that you be careful to water them at least every two days for when they are small they want water frequently."

POTATO POULTICE

Since ancient times, poultices have been considered one of the most effective ways of applying healing substances to the human body, and vegetable poultices especially are an old-time American favorite. But here in this western state, in the early years of its settlement, the potato was so much more commonly used in poultices than any other vegetable that it was easy for Californians to believe they'd been first to discover that warm grated raw potatoes applied to an ailing human body were somehow healing. The truth is that early California poultice makers used this homey old vegetable more often than they did others simply because it was so much more readily available. Along with Chili Pepper, Onions, and beans, it was found in every garden from one end of the land to the other.

According to many prominent herbalists, poultice makers (in California or anywhere else) couldn't do better than choose this most dependable of all "kitchen remedies," one that's long been touted as a boon to victims of rheumatic pains, itches, minor burns, and bruises of every variety.

The potato poultice is still used by some Californians today, not only the rural oldtimers whom one might expect to dip into the vegetable bin for remedies, but younger residents too, like Casey Moneymaker, a Santa Rosa housewife and mother of six, who often turns to old-fashioned remedies to treat her family's minor aches and pains.

QUININE

Cinchona pubescens

The curative powers of the bitter bark of the Quinine tree were discovered by Spanish Jesuit priests in the Andes mountains of South America in the seventeenth century. For several years after its discovery, widespread hatred of the Jesuits caused the substance itself to remain in disuse. Ultimately, however, it was so badly needed—especially for the treatment of the deadly malaria—that it met with acceptance and came to be regarded as the miracle drug of the nineteenth century. The word "Quinine" was on the lips of every early settler, but the remedy itself was often in short supply. Residents were always on the lookout for native medicinal plants that might serve as its substitute.

RICE WATER

In early California, especially during the gold rush era, rice water was common fare for the sick and convalescing, often the only substance that "saddleback doctors" thought fit to pass their lips. Men prepared it for wives recovering from difficult childbirth. Mothers spooned it into the mouths of their ailing offspring. Peter Decker mixed some up and fed it to a fellow forty-niner who'd succumbed to the hazards of an era known as the "sickly season" by those who lived (as Peter did) to tell of its travails.

ROSE GERANIUM

Pelargonium graveolens

Many California settlers, especially those who made the trip westward in the early twentieth century, brought their potted Geraniums along with them when they came. It seemed the right thing to do. After all, the cheery-looking, prettily-scented *Pelargonium* ranked right along with the castiron doorstop, the rooster in the dooryard, and the cat on the hearth when it came to making a house a home.

Most beloved of all the *Pelargoniums*, perhaps—and one of several Geraniums that happens to have earned a reputation as a medicinal herb—is the nose-beguiling Rose Geranium. Jean Heather Darsey of Three Rivers, California, is just one of countless Californians whose childhood memories include encounters with this plant. When she was a youngster suffering from an earache, her mother's housekeeper carefully placed crushed Rose Geranium leaves in her ear, propped a padded hot water bottle against her head, and, in Jean's own words ". . . within an hour, magically . . . no more earache!" She has more to say on the subject. "This has been a family remedy ever since," she declares, and goes on to add ". . . my 'ear-ache plant' is worth its weight in gold when an emergency arises!"

Modern aroma therapists might argue that the only curative value of the Rose Geranuim is its scent, but even this seems more of an endorsement than a debunking.

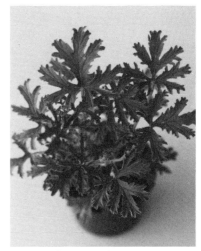

Rose Geranium

ROSEMARY

Rosemarinus officinalis

This historic medicinal plant, favorite of the old world gypsies, prime ingredient of "The Queen of Hungary's Water," pride of the Arabs, and panacea of the Spanish peasants, was grown in California gardens as early as 1826, especially around Santa Barbara, which was for a time the only place that it could be obtained. Then (as for many years before and after) the herb was used as a hair tonic, an insecticide, a heart remedy, a headache treatment, a good luck charm, a cure for insomnia, and an insurance against nightmares. It was a treatment for female complaints, impure blood, obesity, weak liver, wounds, and falling hair.

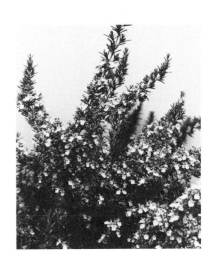

Rosemary

RUE

Ruta graveolins

This herb was cultivated in several early California gardens, those at the missions as well as private plots like that of Don Jose M. de Estudillo. As difficult as it was for a Californio to obtain garden tools in those days—so difficult that Don Ignacio Martinez sent all the way to Hawaii to beg a shipment of Mattock hoes—herb lovers always found a way to plant and cultivate their favorite medicinals. Dangerous though it was (and still is), capable of producing nerve derangement in cases of overdose, Rue was unquestionably one of those favorites. A Rue tea was said to be a good nervine, a Rue ointment an excellent salve for sore joints, gout, and sciatica.

TEA

Early settlers had almost as much faith in black tea as they did in black coffee, and served it often to the sick and the dying. Gold miners especially seemed to have an almost superstitious faith in the curative powers of these two common beverages.

WINE

In 1843 there lived in southern California a certain Frenchman, a gentleman by the name of Louis Vignes, who grew the first oranges in Los Angeles, produced the finest wine in all the land, foretold the future as to the prospect of both of these pursuits, and convinced many of his peers that wine was medicinal. According to William Heath Davis, Jr., who admired the man as much as he did his wine (which he said could be drunk with impunity), Vignes ought to have won the title of the father of the California wine industry. "It is to be hoped," Davis wrote, "that historians will do justice to his character, his labors and foresight."

As it happened, the hopes of Davis were in vain; history hasn't done Louis Vignes justice at all. But Vignes did do *wine* justice; about this there is no question. An altruistic sort, he even gave it to the poor and convinced them in the process that they needed it almost as much as they needed food. As Davis put it ". . . in their distress he helped them in bread, money, and wine. When they came to him he advised the mothers of young children to give them a little wine as an internal antiseptic, so that they might grow up strong, as in his own country; or on the same principle, perhaps, that doctors prescribe whiskey and milk as a cure for diptheria."

This old vintner's peers paid him more heed than history has, for the land's early residents firmly believed there was nothing better for them than a glass of good California wine, especially if it hailed from the vineyard of Vignes.

WINTER SAVORY

Satureja montana

Here was another old-country herb, a native of the Mediterranean region, and a very fragrant plant much-prized by the early Californians. It was grown in the Spaniards' gardens, on the mission grounds, and in the dooryards of latter day settlers, and commonly used as a remedy for gas pains, as a general tonic, and as an antiseptic gargle.

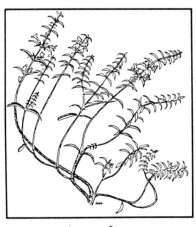

Winter Savory

5
Non-Vegetal Remedies of Old California

Ants. It was a custom of the Chukchansi Indians to treat their stomach aches with a particularly potent counterirritant: a "poultice" of live ants applied liberally to the ailing abdomen. Drastic as it sounds today, this was not an unusual sort of treatment in early California. Ants were perceived by several tribes as both the cause of some diseases and the cure of others. Consider the Luiseno Indians of southern California. These natives had a ceremony, actually an agonizing testing ordeal for boys entering manhood, which they called *Antish*, a word meaning "anting" or "red ant." At this event the young men were either laid atop ant hills or let down into holes that were literally crawling with these little red warriors. Once properly positioned there, the boys were made to remain until they'd suffered their quota of bites and stings. Ultimately, the ants were whipped from their smarting bodies, but ironically, they were beaten away with whips devised from the foliage of the Stinging Nettle plant, which, of course, only caused more pain in the process.

The *Antish* was obviously intended, at least in part, as an endurance test, a way the youths could show their mettle, prove their worth, and establish their manhood. But it may have been a curative rite as well, a purging session during which the young men were rid of whatever incipient maladies might have been ailing them at the time—not to mention those that might have stricken them in later life had they not been stung.

Bitter Medicine. To the California Indians, as to many other native Americans, bitter medicine was oftentimes considered the best medicine of all. Wise counsel to a Luiseno girl generally included this admonition: ". . . when you are pregnant you will drink bitter medicine."

Bloodletting. The shamans of the Chukchansi tribe used to incise cuts between the eyes of patients suffering from headache and sleepwalking.

Curses. Most California Indians believed in the power of their shamans to place disease or death-causing curses on their enemies if they so desired. In some tribes, the shaman was perceived to be just as much a curser as he was a healer. Both feared and beloved, he was at once a danger and a salvation.

Dreams. Nearly all the Indians of California placed great significance on the dreams of their shamans, many of whom claimed to have first learned of their shamanistic prowess from the insightful messages that came to them as they slept. Later on, some of them could even enact cures by their dreaming, just as they could by their singing, their dancing, or their incantation of a fitting formula. Because this was so, most Indians put great stock in the psychic states of their medicine men. But to Mojaves, the art of inner imaging and the ability to learn, grow, and heal, in and through the act of dreaming, was the gift and the duty of every member of the tribe. It was even more important to them than the ritual singing of their mythic songs, their repitious formulas, and epic tales that lent the world its shape and form. "Sumakwanga, Sunakahuwam," they would sing, "Dream, dream." And dream they did, in such a way that there was a sense that every Mojave was his or her own shaman. This is not to say that they had no special medicine men, for they did indeed. These were the chosen ones, the especially gifted singers and dreamers, hand-picked and given healing powers by the god, Mastamho. But every member of the tribe was an inveterate dreamer. Dreams were the very fabric of their lives. A Mojave who didn't dream would not only have been a sick Indian, he probably would have died of a kind of spiritual malnutrition.

Fertility Springs. Childless women—Indians and early settlers alike—sometimes traveled many footweary miles to reach a miraculous northern California spring, the waters of which were said to put an end to barrenness, to insure fertility, to bless with the offspring she desired any longing wayfarer who reached it. Few Californians doubted the beneficence of this freshet; they hardly dared to, for it seemed to them that the proof was all around them in the form of chortling toddlers, proud fathers, and mothers crooning lullabies. Even the sophisticated William Heath Davis, Jr., was a staunch believer, and one who admitted it unabashedly. "Near the presidio," he claimed, "about three-quarters of a mile southeast from the barracks in the grounds of the Miramontes family, was a very remarkable spring called 'Polin'—an Indian name. The spring was long-celebrated for its virtues, which were handed down from the Indians for several generations, and afterward through the Californians. It is claimed that it possessed the remarkable power of producing fecundity in women who were childless and who partook of its waters. Many authentic instances could be quoted in support of this assumption." He went on to mention a few of those who'd left their living testimonials behind them, influential people like Mrs. William D. M. Howard, a San Franciscan of considerable repute, and the good Mrs. Miramontes herself, who bore a total of twenty children, all thanks due, of course, to the precious waters of Polin.

Laying On of Hands. When a Mojave Indian was ill, it meant that his soul, his "shadow," had been stolen away from him, and he needed the services of a shaman to be whole again. Often this healer would sing a series of songs that would make him well, or breathe upon the victim in a certain way, but sometimes the cure was executed by a laying on of hands not unlike that of a modern Christian healer.

Massage. The Diegueno Indian shaman, the *Kwasiyai*, who was destined to be a healer from the moment of birth, sometimes resorted to kneading and pressing, a kind of massage, to cure the sick.

Mud. Ultimately exposed for the imposter that he was, "Doctor" Joe Meeks, who began to practice his dubious brand of medicine in California in 1843, had wrought a few interesting cures before his trickery was discovered. When a bonafide surgeon who sailed into port one day on an American man-of-war cornered him with medical questions that rent him speechless, it was easy enough to debunk Meek's credentials. However, it was not so easy to debunk his cures, especially one that was so impressive that California's governor, Micheltorena, was moved by it to employ him as the official surgeon. (When the sham was discovered, he was discharged, of course, and departed the land forever.) In this memorable case, the medicament that the good "doctor" employed was simply mud: common ordinary California mud. Or so it appeared to those who observed him treating a boy whose toe had been accidentally severed. Meeks stuck the toe back on and bound it with a poultice of nothing other than that homely substance, wet soft earth. The foot healed completely; the toe was sound; the boy was whole. And no one knew how to explain the phenomenon.

Could it be that this notorious imposter knew some secret about the mud he used in that poultice, something of its properties not apparent to the populace in general? Had he discovered a special kind of soil, perhaps something like the Redmond Clay that certain herb dealers tout today? Or had he studied under some Indian shaman who had shown him how to seek and find soil that possessed certain healing ingredients? It's an interesting conjecture, and one that leads toward the consideration of yet another. It's known, for example, that centuries ago, the Egyptians used wet soft earth as a poultice for the stubborn sores and ulcers from which they suffered. It's proposed by some herbalists today that the mud those ancients used may have possessed certain antibiotic properties.

We may never know whether the remarkable "Dr." Meeks learned his muddy secret from Indian shamans or not. But it is a fact that several California tribes did use this substance in at least one medicinal concoction, a pack made of mud and Mesquite-tree sap applied to the human head to rid it of vermin. Perhaps the mud was nothing more than a binder for the sap, perhaps not.

The Costanoan Indians, one-time residents of the San Francisco Bay region, had another use entirely for "Dr." Meeks' favorite medicament. To them it was not a poultice, not a cure-all, an early-day antibiotic, or a vermin killer, but rather simply a protection against the elements, a way to ward off colds, coughs, and chattering teeth. In fact, unlikely though it may seem, it comprised the chilly-weather garb of the men in the tribe, who much preferred to go naked when the weather was seemly. On those chilly, foggy mornings so typical to northern California, these ingenious natives would coat their bodies with common mud and leave it on, like a scuba diver's suit, until the sun came shining through the mist.

Singing. It is said that the Chukchansi Indian shamans could kill with their songs.

Sweat Bath. Promoting spiritual growth, ritual cleansing, improved health, shamanistic insights, good fellowship, visions, devotions, and diversion, the sweat bath was an integral part of the lives of almost all California Indians. Of course it was a practice often misunderstood by non-Indian observers, men whose judgment on native activities was doubtless often preconceived. Even the liberal-minded journalist, Edwin Bryant, who came to California shortly before the gold rush, looked askance at this beloved tribal custom. "The 'sweat-house' is the most important medical agent employed by these Indians," he wrote. "I do not doubt, the effect of consigning many of them to their graves, long before their appointed time."

Despite his negative conclusion, Bryant did give a rather thorough, albeit distinctly biased, description of the sweat house. It was, he said "an excavation in the earth, to the depth of six or eight feet, arched over with slabs split from logs. There is a single small aperture or skylight in the roof. These slabs are covered to the depth of several feet with earth. There is a narrow entrance, with steps leading down and into this subterraneous apartment. Rude shelves are erected around the walls, upon which the invalids repose their bodies. The door is closed and no air is admitted except from the small aperture in the roof, through which escapes the smoke of a fire kindled in the centre of the dungeon. This fire heats the apartment until the perspiration rolls from the naked bodies of the invalids in streams. I incautiously entered one of these caverns during the operation above described, and was in a few moments so nearly suffocated with the heat, smoke, and impure air, that I found it difficult to make my way out."

Notably, there were a few nineteenth-century visitors to sweat houses whose reactions differed considerably from Bryant's. In fact, a member of the famed Lewis-Clark expedition—William Bratton, by name—was cured of terrible back pains and rheumatic stiffness by availing himself of a sweat bath treatment, doubtless quite similar to the one that Bryant berated so roundly.

6
How to be a "Remedy Grower"—Landscaping and Gardening with California's Old-Time Remedies

GETTING STARTED

"Remedy gardening" is a unique pursuit and one that new devotees approach from a wide variety of backgrounds and interests of which, ironically, a life-long love of plants is only one. Here come new residents who simply want their yards to "look western;" here come veteran gardeners of every variety; here come avid wild-food cooks, history buffs, herbalists and collectors of "live antiques." Here too come survivalists, backpackers, nutritionists, folklorists, collectors of Californiana, health food addicts, primitivists, Native Americans exploring their roots, and people involved in holistic health.

Of course, whatever your original motivation, by the time you've decided to engage in remedy gardening or remedy landscaping, you've already fallen in love with plants. Be sure to respect them too. Never make the mistake of digging them up from their own habitat for the sake of a private garden. It's unethical, and in many cases illegal, to remove wildflowers, herbs, shrubs, or trees from the location where they're growing uncultivated and transplant them to your own premises. To do so could indicate a disrespect for plants, disregard for the environment, and disdain for other people.

To gather seeds is an entirely different matter. If the number collected from a perennial plant is small in proportion to the number available, its population will not be affected significantly by the absence of those few. In this case, obviously, it's all right to gather them, assuming, of course, that property owners have granted permission beforehand. Since annuals can only reproduce themselves by seed, theirs should only be collected when it's quite abundant. (Of course seeds can also be purchased from commercial producers, and this is a method of acquiring them that should not be neglected.)

147

When you read in the following section that a plant may be propagated by division of the rhizome, as is the case with the Douglas Iris, this doesn't mean that you should go out into the wilderness, dig up wild Iris plants at random, divide their rhizomes and take them home to plant in your own garden. It does indicate, however, that once you have a Douglas Iris, which you may have purchased at a nursery, found growing on your own property, or acquired through a friend, you may propagate more in this manner.

As to acquiring cuttings, these too should come from your own plants or from those growing on the property of a friend or acquaintance who's willing to share his or her wealth in old medicinals. Never trespass. Never take a plant, a seed, or a cutting without permission. Always remember that an ill-gotten garden can never be a source of pride.

If all this makes it sound as though it's a formidable task to get your garden going, don't you believe it. In some cases getting started is surprisingly easy. The town where you live could be blessed with a commercial nursery featuring medicinal plants and herbs. Or, like tiny Fulton in northern California, it might even boast a nursery that specializes in native California flora. Some cities have chapters of the California Native Plant Society that hold annual California native plant sales where all kinds of treasures can be purchased at a reasonable cost.

Even if it takes a lot of time and energy to find the plants you want to get your remedy garden going, it'll never be a chore. You'll find it an exciting adventure every step of the way. You'll enjoy the jaunts you take to collect your seeds, the new plants you learn about, and all the people you meet who are willing and eager to help you get started. Become a plant detective. Keep your eyes and ears open wherever you go. You'll be surprised at what you find and the fun you have in finding it.

The following are just a few of the many old California remedies that you can grow in your remedy garden. Some of these have been included because they're particularly useful, or beautiful, or adaptable; others are here because they rank among the easiest to start from seeds or cuttings; still others are chosen simply because they're particular favorites of the author. (Be sure to turn back to the field guide section of the book for more details about these old medicinal plants.) Don't stop with these, however. They're only starters. Let your garden grow, and grow, and grow. That's what it's all about.

ALDER

Alnus oregona

Its features. This grand old medicinal tree, the most important hardwood in the state, is valuable for its handsome foliage and its flowers, and not only graces the landscape, but improves the quality of the soil in which it grows. The tree is upright, branching, has a spread of twenty to thirty feet and ranges in height from 100 to 130 feet. It's a very fast-growing tree and will need some pruning and shaping in its youth.

Environment and propagation. The Alder flourishes in a humid climate at altitudes that range from sea level to 2,500 feet. In its wild state it often takes up residence along one of California's many stream beds. It does well in sandy soil, gravel, or clay, but prefers well-drained loam or loamy sand. Easy to start from either seed or cutting, *Alnus oregona* likes constant moisture in the beginning and germinates best in full sunlight.

ANGELICA

Angelica Hendersonii

Its features. Few people would call this coastline-loving plant a beauty. It's a hefty westerner, with an overstuffed look and big bold umbels that could pass as clusters of undersized ping pong balls. But it's an interesting old medicinal, a curiosity, and one that played such a vital role in the folk medicine of early California that it deserves a place of honor in any remedy garden.

This is a towering giant, sometimes reaching as high as six feet, so you'll want to choose its location with the utmost care.

Environment and propagation. Some residents of California's coastal towns and villages consider the Angelica an eyesore and seek to eradicate it from their property. If you already know or chance to meet such a person, he or she will doubtless be delighted if you offer to remove a plant or two. Young plants will transplant quite well. If the foliage dies, don't despair; more will probably sprout up soon. Once you have one plant in your possession, and it's well established and big enough that its root can be divided, you can multiply your wealth. Dust the root with a commercial rooting hormone, divide it, and plant the pieces in desired locations. This can be done at any time of the year.

This hardy westerner can also be started from freshly dried seeds planted in the fall with a very thin cover.

Angelica thrives in a fog belt, likes moist, rich, and well-drained soil, and an open location.

BLUE VERVAIN

Verbena hastata

Its features. Most species of Verbena are at least passably attractive; some are truly showy and make excellent long-blooming garden flowers.

Environment and propagation. These plants do best in a rather poor and sandy soil.

Propagation of the various species of Verbena is either by springtime root division or fall-planted seeds. These plants self-seed nicely, spread widely, and do justice to any California garden.

BORAGE

Borago officinalis

Its features. The wonderful star-like, electric-blue flowers of the Borage make up in beauty for all that's lacked by the coarse-looking foliage. These lovely blooms are as beloved to humankind as they are to the bees who swarm around them endlessly. The plant itself, an annual, generally grows to a height of one and a half to two feet, but in good rich soil may be five feet or even taller.

Environment and propagation. In full sun or partial shade, Borage does best in average garden soil. It's a hardy plant, however, and often thrives in poor, dry soil as well.

Borage transplants poorly, but grows well from seed and self-sows with a vengeance.

CALIFORNIA BUCKEYE

Aesculus californica

Its features. Although its foliage is short-lived, this native deciduous tree is one of California's real beauties, as beloved by today's residents as it was by the Indians to whom it was a source of both food and medicine. It's big, palmately compound leaves are eye-catching themselves, and the pale pinkish flowers, which hang in lush, drooping panicles, are absolutely stunning. A good shade tree, broad and handsome, of variable shape, and ranging in height from fifteen to forty feet, the Buckeye does well on slopes and is a good plant for erosion control. Its growth rate is moderate.

Environment and propagation. This much-prized westerner prefers cool coastal areas, full sun or partial shade, and altitudes under 5,000 feet.

The California Buckeye can be started from either seeds or cuttings.

CALIFORNIA POPPY

Eschscholzia californica

Its features. No California flower garden should be without the state flower, the bright and lovely, historically important and happily long-blooming California Poppy. Early Spanish settlers called it *Copa de oro*, "cup of gold," and aptly so, for it's as golden as a nugget, cup-shaped, cheering, and it's easy to grow.

Environment and propagation. As long as it's planted in a sunny location where the soil is well-drained, the California Poppy is content almost anywhere. It seems to do as well in gardens as it does along roadsides, in fields, and in vacant lots.

This is a protected plant. Don't pull one up and transplant it. It can't abide uprooting and would probably only die anyway. Start your garden poppies from good commercial seeds planted ⅛–¼ inch deep—in the precise location where you want them to grow.

CHICORY

Chichorium intybus

Its features. Despite its attractive flowers of summer-sky blue, Chicory has become such a common roadside plant in California, such a hardy wilding and so apt to crop up in places where it's uninvited that it's thought of more often as a weed than as the worthwhile plant it really is. Open-minded plant lovers, however, find it an asset to the herb garden.

Environment and propagation. Chicory likes rich soil and full sun.
  This herb starts well from seeds planted in late spring or mid-summer.

COMFREY

Symphytum asperum

Its features. Practically every self-respecting herb gardener in the state of California, or any place else, for that matter, has at least one Comfrey plant growing in the dooryard. This is true in spite of the fact that it's rarely considered exceptionally attractive. Its stems are bristly; its leaves are big and coarse and quick to wilt; its curving clusters of purplish flowers are so small compared to its giant foliage that they sometimes go unnoticed. Still, when it comes to old standbys, this herb shines too brightly to be dismissed.

Environment and propagation. Thriving especially in well-drained, moist, moderately rich loam, Comfrey will grow in almost any soil that's not left unwatered. A fast grower, happiest in partial shade, it's an easy plant to get started and a difficult one to stop. One root can be dug up, divided into a dozen pieces, each part replanted, and *voila*—up come ten or twelve more Comfrey plants, enough to make poultices for an army of herbalists.

DIGGER PINE

Pinus sabiniana

Its features. Even among its most ardent fans, there are few Californians who'd rate the Digger as the loveliest of pines. It lacks the typical pine tree shape; its color is dull; the shade it casts is puny. Still, in some ways and in some places it's a most desirable tree. Reaching heights that range from 40 to 60 feet, it's a rapid grower; it controls erosion; it's an excellent windbreak.

Environment and propagation. The Digger Pine tolerates full sun, and arid locations suit it fine, as do gravel and shallow soil. It'll flourish with little water and little care, but give it rich, moist soil and it'll thank you with even faster growth.

This unprepossessing native can be started from either seeds or cuttings.

DOGWOOD

Cornus nuttallii

Its features. One of the best known trees in the country, beloved wherever it grows, the Dogwood needs no advertisement. With its green flowerheads, its pure white petal-like bracts, and its fruit of red drupes, there's no more ornamental plant in the land. A slow-growing tree that rarely needs pruning, the Dogwood will grow to a height of thirty feet.

Environment and propagation. The Dogwood likes a temperate climate, and partial shade at altitudes that range from 200 to 6,000 feet. Growing wild, it favors moist slopes and bottom lands. Strive to duplicate this environment wherever you plant it and it should do well.

The Pacific Dogwood may be started from either seeds or cuttings, set out in moist, well-drained soil.

DOUGLAS IRIS

Iris douglasiana

Its features. This delicate-looking wilding is as favored by California rock gardeners as it is by the bees to whom it's most certainly beloved. The flowers, which are generally blue, can range in hue from pale buff to reddish-purple. It's not an easy plant to cultivate, but so beautiful that it's well worth the effort.

Environment and propagation. The Douglas Iris much prefers light shade, and moist, well-drained soil rich in organic matter.

The plant is best propagated by division of its rhizome after flowering time. First cut the leaves back to a length of about five inches. Then separate between the tufty clumps. These segments should be planted barely below the surface of the soil, about nine inches apart.

DOUGLAS FIR

Pseudotsuga menziesii

Its features. This native evergreen, best known for its excellent lumber, makes a good windbreak, a fine Christmas tree, and a handsome contribution to many a California yard. A rapid grower, it ranges in height from 70 to 250 feet, sometimes even taller. When young, it may need some pruning to keep it compact, but after that it's usually on its own, a good-looking tree with a pyramidal shape and long drooping branches.

Environment and propagation. The Douglas Fir likes a humid environment, good drainage, full sun or partial shade, altitudes below 5,000 feet, and plenty of water.

Most people successfully start this deep-rooted tree from cuttings set in well-draining soil.

ELDERBERRY

Sambucus caerulea

Its features. With its plump clusters of creamy-white flowers and showy bunches of enticing berries, the Blue Elderberry is appreciated just as much today as it was in the nineteenth century when every roving newcomer to set foot in California rhapsodized at length over its abundance of delicious edible berries.

A worthwhile addition to any California landscape, the Blue Elderberry can serve as a good visual screen and a windbreak as well. It can be a rapid and rampant grower, however, and will probably need some thinning now and again.

Variably shaped, considered a large shrub or a small tree, the Blue Elderberry ranges in height from 15 to 30 feet and is sometimes as wide as it is tall.

Environment and propagation. The Blue Elderberry favors full sun or partial shade and altitudes as high as 10,000 feet. Under cultivation it will do best in light, moist, well-drained soil.

This tree can be started well from cuttings. Use light, moist soil.

EVENING PRIMROSE

Oenothera hookeri

Its features. The showy Evening Primrose is a true beauty, sometimes a mid-sized plant, three feet tall, sometimes a towering giant (an occasional specimen reaching as high as nine feet!), a wonderful old medicinal plant, and a cheering addition to any garden.

Environment and propagation. This plant wants ample room, full sun, and moist soil. Some gardeners claim it does well in moderately dry soil as well, but after having seen it thriving in the wilds in marshy locations and in her own back yard, where it's watered almost daily, the author would never advise a dry habitat for the handsome Evening Primrose.

Propagate this plant from seeds, which may be scratched into the soil in either the spring or the fall, and kept moist thereafter.

GOOSEBERRY

Ribes californicum

Its features. A perfect ornamental, with its drooping peduncles of showy crimson flowers, this old medicinal plant is useful too as a background plant, a barrier, and a source of fine edible berries—especially good in pies. The Gooseberry ranges in height from three to ten feet. Its growth is from moderate to rapid and it requires little pruning.

Environment and propagation. The Gooseberry fares well with plenty of moisture and partial shade, at altitudes that range from sea level to 2,000 feet.
   In moist, well-drained soil, the plant can be started from either seeds or cuttings.

LAUREL

Umbellularia californica

Its features. This fine tree, favorite of the Indians and early settlers alike, is cherished by many modern Californians too. They seem not to mind that it needs periodic thinning, that it produces a lot of litter, and that it's prone to unattractive sucker growth. For the ready availability of its multipurpose leaves if for no other reason, cooks and medicinal plant enthusiasts especially delight in the sight and scent of this aromatic tree. Rapid-growing, excellent for shade, this tree sometimes reaches a height of 80 feet.

Environment and propagation. This aromatic tree of canyons and valleys below 5,000 feet does well in full sun or partial shade and is tolerant to weather and wind. As a landscape specimen it will do best in moist and fertile well-drained soil. Get it started from either seeds (that have first been cracked) or cuttings.

MADRONE

Arbutus menziesii

Its features. An evergreen, the Madrone is a splendid tree and a colorful one with its dark green foliage, its fragrant, waxy-white flowers (shaped like little urns), and its sherry-colored bark. Its shape is variable; sometimes it's shrubby and short; sometimes quite sizable—as tall as 100 feet. It's not a fast grower, but at any size it's an easy-care tree, a true beauty and an asset to any landscape.

Environment and propagation. Although it favors warm, rather moist locations, and finds a fog belt beneficial, the Madrone can tolerate a variety of climatic conditions including drought. Start it from cuttings in moist sandy soil.

MANZANITA

Arctostaphylos manzanita

Its features. Anyone striving for natural landscaping, for a woodsy flavor and a country air, can certainly achieve these ends with the fascinating Manzanita shrub. With its tortured branches, its burgundy-colored bark, and its bright red berries, this "Little Apple" of the early Spanish settlers is as charmingly rustic-looking as an old weathered well pump. Although many Californians refer to this plant as a tree, and it's true that an occasional specimen may exceed its own bounds and grow as tall as forty feet, it's really classified as a shrub and usually behaves accordingly.

Environment and propagation. This old westerner is tough, able to tolerate all kinds of weather and all kinds of soil, at altitudes that range from sea level to 5,000 feet. Once established, it's an easy-care plant, but it's not easy to get a Manzanita started. The feat is best accomplished in the fall of the year by transplanting root crowns into soil that's both rich and sandy. If all else fails, look for a nursery that carries Manzanita seedlings.

OUR LORD'S CANDLE

Yucca whipplei

Its features. It was the early Spanish padres who gave this remarkable south-westerner its most poetic name: Our Lord's Candle—an inspired moniker prompted, no doubt, by its great, straight spike of sweet-scented white flowers that rises up toward the sky like a giant taper. Its second most common name, Spanish Bayonet (doubtlessly bequeathed by someone who happened to bump up against its lethal-looking sword-pointed leaves) is considerably less romantic but equally fitting. A study in opposites, a lesson in contradictions, a fascinating symbol of America's far southwest, Our Lord's Candle is a favorite ornamental in many a California yard and garden.

Environment and propagation. There's no need to chill the seeds of Our Lord's Candle, but it's a good idea to soak them in water for a couple of days prior to their autumn planting. Place them in well-draining soil at a depth of about one-half inch. Seedlings should be thinned and placed about five feet apart. The plant needs lots of space, plenty of water in the winter, dry soil in the summer.

PENSTEMON

Penstemon spectabilis

Its features. The Showy Penstemon is as interesting as it is beautiful. The beauty lies in its inflated, tubular flowers, which have the good grace to bloom during the first year of the plant's life. These range in color from blue to purplish to rosy pink. The interest is piqued by its foliage, for the Penstemon's coarsely-toothed, bright-green leaves are borne in pairs that clasp the stem as if they're hanging on in desperation. A fine old medicinal plant, it's an instant eye-catcher.

Environment and propagation. This fascinating wild flower fares the best in sunny locations in a soil that's exceptionally well-drained. It can sometimes tolerate shade, but never constant moistness.

The best way to propagate Showy Penstemon plants is by seeds. These should be scratched—just barely—into the surface of the soil and kept moist until the seedlings are well established. (After they've got a good start however, be careful not to overwater.)

You can also propagate this plant by root division, preferably in the late fall. Divide the rootstock, making sure that each separate division has a shoot bud intact and that it's planted with that bud just at the surface of the soil.

PRICKLY POPPY

Argemone spp.

Its features. Some southwesterners regard this plant as a pesky poisonous weed. To others—like the author—it's one of the most beautiful wild flowers in California. True, its foliage is as prickly as its name implies; it's hard to handle; it's not one you'll pick and put in a vase. But its papery white bloom is absolutely exquisite, a feast to the eye of whomsoever roams through the remedy garden where it grows.

Environment and propagation. In its natural state, the Prickly Poppy is content on the arid desert, keeping company with plants like Jimson Weed, Joshua Tree, and the Creosote Bush. Likewise, in the remedy garden it'll thrive in dry, sandy, or gravelly soil in the sunniest spot you can find. It's easy to propagate. Plant the seeds in the spring of the year, at a depth of about ⅛ inch, in the spot you've picked as a permanent location.

WILD GINGER

Asarum spp.

Its features. This enchanting woodland plant with heart-shaped leaves that look like valentines (and are regarded with the same eye to romance), makes a peerless ground cover and is a distinct asset to anyone's remedy garden. Its flowers are unusual: purplish-brown, minus petals, and, like love notes tucked away in secret, hidden from view by the leaves.

Environment and propagation. Wild Ginger is a woodland dweller and a lover of shade and moisture. Find a place in your remedy garden that follows this description and it'll do quite well.

If you have one Wild Ginger plant, you can acquire more of them with just a little time and trouble. In the fall of the year, after the leaves have wilted, divide its creeping rhizome into pieces and plant each of these about one half inch deep in soil to which you've added some rich organic matter. Leave the bud tips just barely beneath the surface of the soil and then mulch the area well with deciduous leaves.

YERBA BUENA

Satureja douglasii

Its features. This remarkably historic member of the mint family is a hardy but dainty-looking vine that forms an attractive ground cover in shady places and makes a deliciously refreshing tea. It was once so beloved to early Californians that its name was attached to the settlement that later grew up to be San Francisco.

Environment and propagation. Yerba Buena is a rapid-growing, fast-spreading, moisture-loving plant, happiest in locations not unlike its wild habitats of ravines, woodlands, or coastal scrub. It tolerates full sun if it's planted right on the coast, but in inland locations fares much better in shade.

In rich, moist soil, this historic old medicinal is easy to propagate from either seeds or cuttings, and since it's a very common California plant, you should have no trouble acquiring either.

7

An Alphabetical List of Ailments and the Names of the Remedies Early Californians Used to Treat Them

Allergy
  Evening Primrose
Anemia
  Rocky Mountain Bee Plant
Appetite, Poor
  Gooseberries
Arthritis
  Big Root
  Blue Gum
  Comfrey
  Death Camas
  Curly Dock
  Digger Pine
  Douglas Fir
  Elderberry
  Hop
  Laurel
  Marsh Marigold
  Nettle
  Our Lord's Candle
  Pine

  Storkbill
  Sweet Clover
  Wild Onion
  Willow
  Wormwood
  Yerba Mansa
  Yerba Santa
Asthma
  Blue Gum
  Comfrey
  Evening Primrose
  Gumplant
  Honeysuckle
  Wild Onion
  Yerba Mansa
  Yerba Santa
Bedwetting
  Uva-Ursi
Bladder Complications
  Gooseberry
  Honeysuckle

Horsetail
Manzanita
Ox-eye Daisy
Uva-Ursi
Western Coltsfoot
Wild Grape
Wild Onion

Breath, Bad
Angelica
Parsley

Bronchial Problems
Barberry
Blue Gum
Gumplant
Marsh Marigold
Mustard
Nettle
Scarlet Lobelia
Uva-Ursi

Bruises
Beavertail
Death Camas
Digger Pine
Dutchman's Pipe
Fremont Cottonwood

Burns and Scalds
Comfrey
Digger Pine
Dutchman's Pipe
Hound's Tongue
Pine
Yerba Mansa

Cancer
Red Clover

Childbirth, Facilitating
Abstinence from salt, meat, and tobacco
  (Mojave Indian)
Alder
Bear's Hair potion supplied by a Chukchansi bear
  doctor
Wake Robin

Colds
Blue Gum
Blue Vervain
Dog Fennel
Elderberry
Evening Primrose
Green Amaranth
Gumplant
Horehound

Madrone
Mallow
Mustard
Peony
Pine
Redbud
Wild Onion
Wild Rose
Woolly Mullein
Yerba Santa

Colic
Blue Gum
Fennel
Lacepod
Pineapple Weed
Yerba Buena

Complexion Problems
Comfrey
Elderberry
Honeysuckle
Pine

Constipation
Cascara Buckthorn
Chicory
Coffeeberry
Curly Dock
Dandelion
Elderberry
Horehound
Licorice
Plantain
Wild Rose

Cough and Congestion
Angelica
Blackberry
Evening Primrose
Gumplant
Licorice
Madrone
Mallow
Mustard
Ox-eye Daisy
Peony
Sweet White Clover
Wild Onion
Wild Rose
Yerba Santa

Cuts and Scratches
Horsetail
Hound's Tongue

Madrone
Marsh Woundwort
Oregon Ash
Plantain
Shepherd's Purse
Wild Ginger
Wild Grape
Wood Sorrel
Yarrow
Yerba Mansa
Yerba Santa

Dandruff, Dry or Lusterless Hair, etc.
Amole
Nettle
Our Lord's Candle

Death Cap Mushroom Poisoning
Milk Thistle

Diarrhea
Goose Grass
Green Amaranth
Groundsel
Horehound
Pineapple Weed
Shepherd's Purse
Wild Grape
Willow

Dropsy
Conchalagua

Epilepsy
Cow Parsnip
Queen Anne's Lace

Eyes, Inflamed, Sore, Itchy, etc.
Angelica
Fennel
Marsh Marigold
Marsh Woundwort
Mesquite
Nightshade
Prickly Poppy
Teasel

Feet, Tired, Sore, etc.
Creosote Bush

Female Complaints
Blackberry
Bracken Tea Licorice
Coast Eriogonum
Hop
Horehound
Manzanita
Nettle

Plantain
Shepherd's Purse
Uva-Ursi
Wake Robin
Wild Rose
Wormwood

Fever
Canchalagua
Dogwood (used as a Quinine substitute)
Elderberry
Gooseberry
Hop
Horehound
Redbud (used as a Quinine substitute)
Turkey Mullein
Willow

Flatulence
Fennel
Mint

Gall Bladder Complications
Creeping Jenny
Dandelion

General Debility
Arrowhead
Blue Vervain
Canchalagua
Clover
Comfrey
Dogwood
Sage
Wake Robin
Yerba Buena

Gout
Blue Vervain
Storkbill

Headache
Alder
Blue Curls
Coast Eriogonum
Cow Parsnip
Cuts incised between the eyes (Chukchansi Indians)
Evening Primrose
Fremont Cottonwood
Laurel
Manzanita
Meadow Rue
Nettle
Willow
Yarrow
Yerba Buena

Hemorrhages
Alder
Goose Grass
Horsetail
Marsh Woundwort
Shepherd's Purse
Uva-Ursi
Yarrow

Insomnia
Blue Vervain
California Poppy
Coffeeberry
Hop
Indian Tobacco (Yurok and other Indians)
Nightshade

Itches
Plantain
Prickly Poppy
Willow

Kidney Problems
Elderberry
Manzanita
Queen Anne's Lace
Uva-Ursi
Western Coltsfoot
Wild Grape
Wood Sorrel

Lactation, Excess
Sage

Lactation, Poor
Chicory
Fennel
Milk Thistle

Laryngitis
Mustard
Sage

Liver Problems
Barberry
Bracken Fern
Creeping Jenny
Milk Thistle

Lung, Weakness, Disease, Congestion, etc.
Alder
Angelica
Bracken
Comfrey
Creosote Bush
Fern
Mustard
Turkey Mullein

Western Coltsfoot
Woolly Mullein
Yarrow
Yerba Mansa
Yerba Santa

Menstrual Irregularities
Blackberry
Bracken Fern
Licorice
Manzanita
Nettle
Plantain
Shepherd's Purse
Uva-Ursi
Wake Robin
Wild Rose
Wormwood

Mental Problems
Coffeeberry
Gumplant

Nausea
Blackberry
Cow Parsnip
Mint
Yerba Buena
Yerba Mansa

Nervousness
Blue Vervain
California Poppy
Coffeeberry
Groundsel
Gumplant
Horehound

Nosebleed
Goose Grass
Shepherd's Purse
Willow

Oral Hygiene
Angelica
California Buckeye
California Nutmeg
California Poppy
Parsley
Wild Rhubarb

Piles
Buffalo Gourd
Goose Grass
Woolly Mullein
Yarrow

Pneumonia
Alder
Angelica
Bracken Fern
Coffeeberry
Creosote Bush
Mustard
Turkey Mullein
Western Coltsfoot
Yerba Mansa

Poison Oak
Amole
Wild Onion

Rattlesnake Bite
Angelica
Dogtooth Violet
Extraction of venom by a Yokut snake shaman
Four specified songs sung by a Mojave shaman
Horehound
Milkweed
Oregon Ash
Plantain
Poison Oak
Wild Grape

Rheumatism
Elderberry
Hop
Laurel
Marsh Marigold
Nettle
Our Lord's Candle
Pine
Storkbill
Sweet White Clover
Wild Onion
Willow
Wormwood
Yerba Mansa
Yerba Santa

Seasickness
Mint

Skin Problems, Rashes, Boils, Pimples, etc.
Figwort
Fremont Cottonwood
Giant Blazing Star
Groundsel
Honeysuckle
Larkspur
Manzanita
Our Lord's Candle

Penstemon
Pine
Plantain
Prickly Poppy
Shepherd's Purse
Squaw Bush
Teasel
Wild Grape
Willow
Wood Sorrel
Yerba Mansa

Sleepwalking
Patient cut between the eyes by a Chukchansi Indian shaman

Smallpox
Squaw Bush

Sore Throat
Angelica
Blackberry
Blue Gum
Blue Vervain
Creosote Bush
Dog Fennel
Licorice
Madrone
Peony
Pine
Wild Onion
Wild Rhubarb

Sores
Blue Vervain
Buffalo Gourd
California Poppy
Castor Bean
Chicory
Comfrey
Death Camas
Digger Pine
Dutchman's Pipe
Figwort
Fremont Cottonwood
Giant Blazing Star
Groundsel
Honeysuckle
Horsetail
Madrone
Manzanita
Penstemon
Pine

Plantain
Yerba Mansa
Splinters
 Comfrey
 Pine Pitch
 Potato Poultice
Sprains
 Death Camas
 Digger Pine
 Dutchman's Pipe
Stings and Bites
 Mallow
 Plantain
 Rocky Mountain Bee Plant
Stomach Ulcers
 Comfrey
Stomach Ache
 Alder
 Angelica
 Barberry
 Blackberry
 Blue Curls
 California Poppy
 Coast Eriogonum
 Dogwood
 Elderberry
 Fennel
 Giant Blazing Star
 Green Amaranth
 Groundsel
 Lacepod
 Laurel
 Madrone
 Mallow
 Mint
 Pigweed
 Pineapple Weed
 Rocky Mountain Bee Plant
 Sage
 Squaw Bush
 Stinging ants applied to ailing stomach (Chukchansi
  Indian)
 Sweet White Clover
 Toyon
 Wood Sorrel
 Yerba Mansa

Swelling
 Chicory
 Comfrey
 Creosote Bush
 Dogtooth Violet
 Mallow
 Sweet White Clover
 Yerba Mansa
 Yerba Santa
Toothache
 Licorice
 Willow Bark
 Woolly Mullein
 Yarrow
Venereal Disease
 Angelica
 Big Root
 Century Plant
 Green Amaranth
 Indian Fig
 Plantain
 Sneezeweed
 Willow
Vermin
 Larkspur
 Laurel
 Mesquite
 Wormwood
Warts
 Poison Oak
 Teasel
Wounds
 Horsetail
 Hound's Tongue
 Madrone
 Marsh Woundwort
 Oregon Ash
 Plantain
 Shepherd's Purse
 Wild Ginger
 Wild Grape
 Wood Sorrel
 Yarrow
 Yerba Mansa
 Yerba Santa

Bibliography

Audubon, John Woodhouse. *Audubon's Western Journal, 1849–1850.* Tucson, Arizona: The University of Arizona Press, 1984. (First Edition, Cleveland Ohio: Arthur H. Clark Company, 1906.)

Angier, Bradford. *Field Guide to Medicinal Wild Plants.* Harrisburg, Pennsylvania: Stackpole Books, 1978.

Art, Henry W. *A Garden of Wildflowers, 101 Native Species and How To Grow Them.* Pownal, Vermont: Storey Communications, Inc., 1986.

Bakker, Elna. *An Island Called California, An Ecological Introduction to Its Natural Communities.* Berkeley and Los Angeles: University of California Press, 1984.

Ball, Edward K. *Early Uses of California Plants.* Berkeley and Los Angeles: University of California Press, 1970.

Barrows, David Prescott. *Ethno-Botany of the Coahuilla Indians.* Banning, California: Malki Museum Press, 1977.

Bean, Lowell John and Saubel, Katherine Siva. *Temalpakh, Cahuilla Indian Knowledge and Usage of Plants.* Morongo Indian Reservation: Malki Museum Press, 1972.

Belzer, Thomas J. *Roadside Plants of Southern California.* Missoula: Mountain Press Publishing Company, 1984.

Bidwell, John. *Life in California Before the Gold Discovery.* Los Angeles: Ward Ritchie Press, 1948. (First published in *The Century Magazine,* Dec. 1890 and February, 1891.)

Bolton, Herbert Eugene, Ph.D. *Kino's Historical Memoir of Primeria Alta, A Contemporary Account of the Beginnings of California, Sonora, and Arizona, by Father Eusebio Francisco Kino, S. J.* Berkeley and Los Angeles: University of California Press, 1948.

Brockman, Frank C. *Trees of North America.* New York: Golden Press, Western Publishing Company, Inc., 1968.

Bryant, Edwin. *What I Saw in California, The Complete Original Narrative and Appendix from the 1849 Appleton Edition, in True Facsimile.* Palo Alto: Lewis Osborne, 1967.

Chestnut, V. K. *Plants Used by the Indians of Mendocino County, California*. Mendocino County: Mendocino County Historical Society, 1974. (First published in Contributions From U.S. National Herbarium, Vol. VII, 1902.)

Coon, Nelson. *Using Plants for Healing, An American Herbal*. Emmaus, Pa.: Rodale Press, 1979.

Crittenden, Mabel and Telfer, Dorothy. *Wildflowers of the West*. Milbrae, California: Celestial Arts, 1975.

Davis, William Heath. *Seventy-five Years in California*. Edited by Small, Harold A. San Francisco, California: John Howell Books. (First published, San Francisco: Andrew J. Leary, 1889.)

Dobelis, Inge N., Dwyer, James, Visallia, Gayla, and other editors. *Magic and Medicine of Plants*. Pleasantville, New York, and Montreal: The Reader's Digest Association, Inc.

Dillon, Richard. *Fool's Gold, The Decline and Fall of Captain John Sutter of California*. Santa Cruz, California: Western Tanager, 1981.

Foster, Steven. *Herbal Bounty, The Gentle Art of Herb Culture*. Salt Lake City: Gibbs M. Smith Inc., Peregrine Smith Books, 1984.

Fuller, Thomas C. and Elizabeth McClintock. *Poisonous Plants of California*. Berkeley, Los Angeles and London: University of California Press, 1986.

Furlong, Marjorie and Pill, Virginia. *Wild Edible Fruits and Berries*. Happy Camp, California: Naturegraph Publishers, 1974.

Garland, Sarah. *The Complete Book of Herbs and Spices*. New York: The Viking Press, 1979.

Gast, Ross H. *Don Francisco de Paula Marin*. (With Conrad, Agnes C., editor. *The Letters and Journal of Francisco de Paula Marin*.) Honolulu: The University Press of Hawaii for the Hawaiian Historical Society, 1973.

Geary, Ida. *The Leaf Book*. Fairfax, California: A. Philpott, The Tamal Land Press, 1972.

Geiger, Maynard, O. F. M. *Franciscan Missionaries in Hispanic California, 1769–1846*. San Marino: The Huntington Library, 1969.

Giff, Helen S., editor. *The Diaries of Peter Decker, Overland to California in 1849 and the Life in the Mines, 1850–1851*. Georgetown, California: The Talisman Press, 1966. (Original Manuscript Diaries in the Collection of Society of California Pioneers, San Francisco.)

Harner, Michael. *The Way of the Shaman*. Toronto, New York, London, Sydney and Auckland: Bantam Books.

Harris, Ben Charles. *Kitchen Medicines, Curative Recipes and Remedies, A Guide to the Pharmacy in Your Kitchen*. New York: Pocket Books, 1973.

Harris, Ben Charles. *The Compleat Herbal*. New York: Larchmont Books, 1975.

Haskin, Leslie L. *Wild Flowers of the Pacific Coast*. New York: Dover Publications, Inc., 1977. (First published, Portland, Oregon: P. Binfords and Mort, 1934.)

Heinerman, John. *The Science of Herbal Medicine*. Orem, Utah: Bi-World Publishers, 1979.

Hutchens, Alma R. *Indian Herbology of North America*. Ontario, Canada: Merco, 1983.

Jepson, Willis Linn. *A Manual of the Flowering Plants of California*. Berkeley, Los Angeles, and London: The University of California Press.

Kastner, Joseph. *A Species of Eternity*. New York: E. P. Dutton. © 1977 by author.

Kirk, Donald R. *Wild Edible Plants of the Western United States*. Healdsburg, California: Naturegraph Publishers, 1970.

Kroeber, A. L. *Handbook of the Indians of California*. New York: Dover Publications, Inc., 1976. (First published by the Government Printing Office, Washington, in 1925.)

Labadie, Emile L. *Native Plants for Use in the California Landscape*. Sierra City, California: Sierra City Press, 1978.

Levy, Juliette de Bairacli. *Common Herbs for Natural Health*. New York: Schocken Books, 1975.

Leyel, Mrs. C. F. *Herbal Delights*. London and Boston: Farber and Farber, 1987. (Printed in Great Britain by Richard Clay Ltd., Bungay, Suffolk.)

Lust, John. *The Herb Book*. Toronto, New York, London, Sydney, Auckland: Bantam Books.

Mabey, Richard. *Plantcraft, a Guide to the Everyday Use of Wild Plants*. New York: Universe Books, 1978.

Margolin, Malcolm. *The Ohlone Way, Indian Life in the San Francisco-Monterey Bay Area*. Berkeley, California: Heyday Books, 1978.

Medsger, Oliver Perry. *Edible Wild Plants*. New York and London: Collier Mac-Millan Publishers, 1974.

Moore, Michael. *Medicinal Plants of the Mountain West*. Sante Fe, New Mexico: The Museum of New Mexico Press.

Munz, Philip A. and Keck, David D. *A California Flora*. Berkeley, Los Angeles and London: University of California Press, 1968.

Munz, Philip A. *California Desert Wildflowers*. Berkeley: University of California Press, 1962.

Munz, Philip A. *California Mountain Wildflowers*. Berkeley and Los Angeles: University of California Press, 1963.

Munz, Philip A. *Shore Wildflowers of California, Oregon and Washington*. Berkeley, Los Angeles, and London: University of California Press, 1964.

Niehaus, Theodore F. and Ripper, Charles L. *Pacific State Wildflowers*. Boston: Houghton Mifflin Company, 1979.

Parsons, Mary Elizabeth. *The Wild Flowers of California, Their Names, Haunts and Habits*. New York: Dover Publications, 1966.

Peterson, Lee Allen. *A Field Guide to Edible Wild Plants*. Boston: Houghton Mifflin Company, 1977.

Potterton, David, editor. *Culpeper's Color Herbal*. New York: Sterling Publishing Co., Inc., 1983.

Powers, Stephen. *Tribes of California*. Berkeley, Los Angeles and London: University of California Press, 1976. (First published 1871.)

Rose, Jeanne. *Herbs and Things, Jeanne Rose's Herbal*. New York: Grosset and Dunlap, Workman Publishing Company, 1979.

Santillo, Humbart. *Natural Healing With Herbs*. Prescott Valley, Arizona: Hohm Press, 1985.

Schmutz, Ervin M. Ph.D. and Hamilton, Lucretia Breazeale. *Plants That Poison*. Flagstaff, Arizona: Northland Press, 1986.

Schultes, Richard Evans. *Medicines From the Earth*. San Francisco: Harper and Row, 1978.

Simpson, Lesley Byrd, translator. *California in 1792, The Expedition of Jose Longinos Martinez.* San Marino, California: Huntington Library Publications, 1938.

Spencer, Edwin Rollin. *All About Weeds.* New York: Dover Publications, Inc., 1975.

Spicer, Edward H., editor. *Ethnic Medicine in the Southwest.* Tucson, Arizona: The Universtiy of Arizona Press, 1979.

Spoerke, David G. Jr. *Herbal Medications.* Santa Barbara, California: Woodbridge Press Publishing Company, 1980.

Tatum, Billy Joe. *Billy Joe Tatum's Wild Foods Field Guide and Cookbook.* New York: Workman Publishing Company, Inc., 1976.

Wagner, Lisa K. *Common Plants of the East Bay, A Guide to Common Non-Woody Plants Found in East Bay Communities.* Berkeley, California: Appletree Press, 1983.

Watts, May Theilgaard. *Master Tree Finder.* New York: Warner Books, 1986.

Wilbur, Marguerite Eyer, editor. *A Pioneer at Sutter's Fort, 1846–1850, The Adventures of Heinrich Lienhard.* Los Angeles: The Calafia Society, 1941.

Index of Scientific Names

Index

Horehound Leaf, 59
Juniper Berry, 71
Lacepod, 71
Laurel Leaf, 74
Manzanita, 80
Mexican, 88
Milkweed, 85
Miner's, 88
Mormon, 69, 79
Nettle, 92
Oak Bark, 94
Our Lord's Candle, 96
Pine Needle, 100
Plantain, 102
Rue, 141
Sage, 107
Shepherd's Purse, 109
Soldier, 58, 59
Squaw, 88
Substitute for Chinese, 15
Sweet Clover, 112
Whorehouse, 88
Wood Sorrel, 124
Teamsters, 89
Teasel, 112
Tehachapi, California, 136
Terrestrial Paradise, 1
Therapist, aroma, 72
Thirst, to quench, 114, 130, 137, 139
Thistle Poppy, 103
Thistle Sage, 106
Thorn Apple, 67
Thousand Seal, 126
Thousand-Leaved, 126
Thread, 63
Three-Leaved Nightshade, 115
Throat, (sore or scratchy), 9, 15, 39, 57, 58, 61, 71, 76, 94, 98
Throats, parched, 114
Tincture, Manzanita, 80
Tobacco, 64–67
Tobacco additive, 126
Tobacco farming
   By Yurok Indians, 66
Tobacco smoking, diagnostic, 66
Tobacco, substitute for, 123
Taboada, Father Luis y, 50
Toloache, 67–69
Toloache rite, 68
Tonics, (from assorted herbs)
   Angelica, 9
   Dogwood, 41
   Grape Wine, 142
   Juniper Berry, 71
   Toyon, 20, 113
Tonics, (for specific purposes)
   Hair, 69, 92, 141

Heart, 63, 135
   Spring, 123
   Stomach, 107, 125
Toothache remedies, 54, 66, 67, 71, 94, 99, 123, 126, 127
Toywort, 108
Trapper, 62
Trebol, 29
Tree Tobacco, 64
Tree, Yucca, 70
Trifoliate, leaves, 4
Trinity County, 40, 51
Trinity Valley, 79
Trinity, Lower, 9
Trout Lily, 40
Tuberculosis, (Consumption), 22, 88, 127, 129, 137
Tubers, 10
Tule Potato, 10
Tuna, 61–63
Turkey Mullein, 16, 113–114
Turpentine Weed, 15
Twine, 63

Ukiah, 65
Ulcers, 22, 86, 89, 97, 107, 116, 129
Umbel, 4
Umbrella Mallow, 77–78
Underarm deodorant, 107
Upland Cranberry, 114
Urinary remedies, 14, 45, 71, 78, 80, 89, 119
Urine, to increase flow of, 11, 53, 62
Utah Juniper, 71
Uterine obstructions, 71
Uva-Ursi, 114–115

Valley White Oak, 93
Vallier, Viola, 27, 134
Velvet Flower, 55
Velvet Plant, 126
Venereal disease, 13, 27, 43, 61, 62, 70, 96, 110, 112
Ventura County, 76
Venus' Basin, 112
Vermin, 84
Vermin killer, 145
Vervain, 17
Viard Indians, 79
Vignes, Louis, 142
Vinegar, 6
Vinegar Weed, 15
Violet, Dogtooth, 40
Violets, 115
Vision, poor, 93

Visions, 146
Vitamin A, 47
Vomiting, 22, 88

Wading, Indian woman, 11
Wailaki Indians, 5–7, 15, 16, 21, 29, 37, 40, 48, 51, 89, 90, 102, 103, 115, 116
Wake Robin, 115–116
Walnut, 95
Warts, 63, 64, 85, 112
Water Birches, 49
Water retention, 80, 111
Water Thistle, 112
Water, emergency drinking, 62
Wax, Myrtle, 41, 102
Way-Bread, 101
Western Bracken, 18, 19
Western Coltsfoot, 116–117
Western Honey Mesquite, 83
Western Peony, 97
Westrich, Jim, 28
White Chenopodium, 98
White Horehound, 58
White House Cook Book, 136
White Sage, 106
White Sweet Clover, 111
White Wood Sorrel, 123
Whitebark Pine, 99
Whitewater Creek, 5
Whiteweed, 96
Whooping Cough, 97
Whorehouse Tea, 98
Wild Anise, 46–47
Wild Bachelor Button, 28
Wild Balsam, 129
Wild Carrot, 104
Wild Cucumber, 13
Wild Currants, 89
Wild Endive, 28
Wild Fuschia, 51
Wild Ginger, 43, 156
Wild Iris, 41
Wild Licorice, 75
Wild Mint, 86
Wild Morning Glory, 33
Wild Teasel, 112
Willows, 5, 20, 95
Wine, 142
Winter Savory, 142–143
Wintun Indians, 79, 88, 133

Yahi Indians, 66
Yarrow, 126–127
Yellow Dock, 35
Yellow Fawn Lily, 40
Yellow Pines, 21, 42, 57, 98, 115